Dr. Paula Hor

Dissolving Co-aependency

Powerful Insights
from the
Core Empowerment Training

LOTUS LIGHT
SHANGRI-LA

1. American Edition 1992
by Lotus Light Publications
P.O.Box 2
Wilmot, WI 53192 USA
The Shangri-La series is published
in cooperation with Schneelöwe Verlagsberatung,
Federal Republic of Germany
Originally published 1991,
© by Schneelöwe Verlagsberatung,
8955 Aitrang, Federal Republic of Germany
All rights reserved

ISBN 0-941524-86-8

Printed in the USA

Acknoledgements

This book was inspired by a need to promote greater understanding of certain concepts which are fundamental to the Core Empowerment Training. Through the course of its development, it became apparent that more time should be spent in experiential work, and less time lecturing on basic principles. In order to condense such an in-depth training into two short weekends, we felt the need to lucidate certain concepts ahead of time and also to provide participants with a prior opportunity to begin self-observation. An introductory evening did not fulfill our needs, thus it seemed imperative to create a book which not only would benefit the reader in daily life, but also would help our participants to be better prepared for the course.

I owe much of the inspiration for this work to Brigitte Ziegler, my partner in this effort, and her uncanny ability to fill in my "blank," spots. Also I would like to acknowledge Don Alexander Riches, our partner, for his support and inspiration in this work and in the development of the training itself.

There are many I would like to credit for their work, which I have previously experienced, and whose ideas are included in both the book and the training: Ken Cadigan, for his work with Charles Berner's Enlightenment Intensive; Doug Morrison for his work with Body Electronics, developed by John Ray; Gabriel Cousins for his great variety of work and ideas; and the various meditation traditions of my two partners Brigitte and Don.

I want to thank my wonderful family for their love and support in this, my most recent endeavor: My sister Patricia for her emotional support; my father for his incredible energy and

3

support in this work by providing me with a quiet place to write, and my sister Kathy for her indomitable efforts at the computer, revising and reworking the English edition of this book and for working in the wee small hours after my two very lovable but feisty nieces were fast asleep, and her husband Rudy for his overall computer expertise.

I must also acknowledge my many wonderful friends (quite a few of whom have been both my students and teachers) around the world for their great inspiration. You have provided me with both the knowledge and support to recognize that conscious awareness is a real possibility on a world scale.

Paula Horan

For about fifteen years I have been intensely involved in the study of human consciousness. During this exploratory journey, I became acquainted with many different tools which helped me to go deeper into the various layers of my mind. I have always been interested in finding techniques which would provide not only "band-aid" style remedies for solving life's problems, but would actually effect very deep changes in consciousness.

During this search, I have been inspired by many teachers and writers to continue my self-work, leading to higher levels of consciousness. I am very grateful for the knowledge I have gleaned from their many insights. I owe a great debt of appreciation to my Zen teachers, who taught me to release most of my mental structures and to live in the moment. Tarthang Tulku's books and exercises also provided a great challenge for helping me to explore parts of the vast unknown regions of my mind. The admirable Sufi master, Irena Tweedie, has further inspired me to follow the path of the heart. With the help of Karl Everding's two year training, I have learned to face the darker aspects of myself, and to commit myself to personal global transformation.

At a crucial and important turning point in my life, I met Paula Horan; her goals, ideas, and experiences on the spiritual path helped me to integrate my own explorations in a wonderful way. Out of a very intense and vibrant cooperation, we developed this book and the present form of the Core Empowerment Training. It was a great challenge and quite a unique experience to write in two languages. Despite all the complications inherent in such a task, the actual writing flowed very well; as we laughed quite often enjoying some of the comical differences between the German and English languages. I want to thank Paula from the bottom of my heart for her power, inspiration and enthusiasm, without which this book would not have developed in such an easy manner. I also want to thank our partner, Don Alexander Riches, whose knowledge and tranquil clarity had a very positive effect on our work.

In addition I would like to recognize all of the people who have accompanied me along my path, and who have touched me deeply and enriched my life and work. I would especially like to acknowledge: my mother, my sister, and my brother for their love and understanding; Brigitta Vedra for her selfless support at a difficult time in my life; and last but not least, my two doctors, Dr. Hermann Mayr and Dr. Johannes Schmidt, who helped me to stand on my own feet in both a literal and figurative sense, after a difficult operation.

Finally, I would like to thank all of our students for their openness, courage, and honesty, and their willingness to face the pain of personal change, which has certainly added to the morphic field of this planet, making it easier for others to follow in their footsteps. To you the reader, I thank you for your willingness to learn and grow, to and
continue on your path to wholeness.

Brigitte Ziegler

Table of Contents

Introduction

We are living in a very exciting period of the earth's history. Severe challenges are upon us - the disruption of old political systems in turn wreaking economic havoc, and the environment screaming out at us to create a major shift in our priorities, are but two of our major concerns. Most of all, what really has greatest priority, is the deep inner calling, the demand as it were, to reckon with the truth of who we are - now. At no time in Earth's history has there been a greater priority. It is indeed time for each one of us to stand up and be counted. All of us must now take full responsibility for our own life condition. We must stop blaming our governments, churches, teachers, bosses, wives, husbands, children, parents, etc. for our "problems." Problems are self-induced, self-created. They are only an illusion. Indeed, life really presents us with only challenges. It is we who turn the challenges into problems by our negative attitude and approach. Whenever we resist what we deem a "negative" situation, we turn it into a problem, for our very resistance fuels the situation with energy. Our greatest challenge in dealing with the "problem" of resistance, is that we are 99% reactive because of thousands of years of conditioning. In addition, most of our resistance is fueled by the ego. It is very difficult to avoid giving back a negative retort, when someone has challenged your ego. The ego generally issues back a barrage of argumentative rhetoric, or rationalizations in a robotic fashion when it is threatened. The true you - the essence of self innocently unattached to being right, gets caught in the cross fire, effectively pinned in the shadow of the ego.

It is high time to loosen ourselves from the grip of the ego, and from the demanding social structures of our time. We must learn from scratch truly to think and act for ourselves from the core-self and to cease reacting to life's various situations in a mechanistic way, as in the blind conditioned response of Pavlov's dog. We must now consider the price of freedom we have so long demanded and given "lip service", but long avoided because of the very terror it evokes in us. True responsibility is a scary propositon for most, who would rather leave life's decisions to someone "smarter" or more experienced. It is easier to "pass the buck" so we can later blame others for our misery. To succumb to the central human computer (Jung's collective unconscious) is the path of least resistance. To follow the demands of society and take your place like a cog in a wheel offers a simple mindless solution. The irony of this path of least resistance is that you eventually find yourself rubbing up against it and robotically resisting life's various situations. The reactivity increases, piling layer upon layer on top of crystallized thought forms, in direct proportion lowering any real possibility of conscious awareness. This is the design of the proverbial rat trap,

one which we have helped create en masse, and a truly difficult one from which to escape.

To become a unique, free thinking, centered individual initially takes a lot of guts and a strong burning desire. Eventually, as we move through our trials with perseverance and discipline, we become naturally self-observant. More and more we begin to catch ourselves in the act of sleep, and in turn steadily develop more conscious awareness. Eventually, we may even become less goal-oriented, as the need for a goal to keep us busy or drive us forward recedes, pervading our everyday lives with a greater sense of being. A natural tendency to do what is right in the moment develops.

Before we can reach a capacity for greater conscious awareness, for being in the moment, a lot of discipline is needed. An understanding of some of our basic mental structures and how they react with emotions is of great importance. The actual creation of thought crystals, the very process of their development within a polarized context, and their effect on consciousness, gives greater insight to the robotic nature of our everyday lives. Such basic knowledge, leading to a greater understanding of the inner working of the mind, is an essential tool for anyone really wishing to be free of the gravity of normal human consciousness. The intention of the authors is to give the reader this basic foundation and, hopefully, to encourage you to use the insights in this book to improve your life condition. This book is also a prerequisite for anyone wishing to partici- pate in the Core Empowerment Training. We encourage you to take your time with the various exercises offered in each chapter, because they will provide you with the personal life experience which is needed to help you benefit more fully from the training. Brigitte, Don and I, wish you great success in your endeavors, and we look forward to meeting many of you in the future.

Paula Horan
Munich

Chapter 1

The Core Self

What is the nature of the essence of self? The true you, the core of the body/mind/spirit, which calls to you, beckons you, to become more truly who you are?

Just who are we? Who is that person who says "I" or "me",and to whom or what does that "I" or "me" refer? Who is it who feels so separated, yet at the same time so identified with everything and everyone else? To try and grasp this mysterious aspect of our being, to gain some insight into this powerful pull we feel, to connect with all that is, we need to look at what it is not.

In the everyday use of the word "I" or "me", we assume that we are talking about one cohesive self. Who we are, seems to be so obvious. Each of us has a body with a certain form, a name, a family, a job, and a story. When we apply for a job or passport, we list all of the essential data without any thought as to who or what we really are. In addition, we tend to identify with certain qualities or traits which we assign ourselves, and receive from the feedback of others. All of these attributes added together seem to lead to the sure or unquestioned belief that we are composed of a certain unified personality - an "I." Very rarely do we question this I, or the image we have of ourselves. Only when we get into trouble does the self image even begin to come into question.

In truth we are composed of many I's. There is the well meaning I who decides to go on a diet, and the I who would rather eat whatever seems appealing in the moment. There is the disciplined I who strongly determined to keep fit, begins a daily exercise routine yet falters when the lazy "I" takes over and decides it would rather sleep. We are constantly faced with a slew of oppositional I's. Thus we can see that the self image which we so cherish and protect is built on quite an unstable foundation. It is composed of a large number of transitory I's, passing through the mind like fleeting images in a dream. When we are identified with one I, all the others seem to pass away - they no longer exist, and we are then totally consumed, indeed hypnotized by the momentary I. In a flash it too may pass away and we are soon absorbed in the needs and desires of the next momentary I.

Everything we identify with changes on both an inner and outer level. The body falls ill, and eventually ages and dies. We may lose our job, our relationship, our family. Over the course of a lifetime we may eventually lose everthing. Nothing remains as it is. Yet in each of us something seems to exist which is not subject to change. It is a kind of inner center - the Core Self.

This Core Self or inner center, which is left behind when all the various identities fall away, is the true essence of self which emanates through all the layers of personality. It is composed of the high vibratory frequency of love energy, as individualized in each unique being. The divine paradox involving the whole description of the Core Self, is that you cannot say of it that it actually does or does not exist. Once you name it, once you say it exists, it becomes a mere thing. In truth it exists beyond time and space; it is not fixed; it cannot be described or even limited within a framework. It is a dynamic vital factor in ourselves which is at the same time both constant and changing. In its pure form it is unbound by the dense energy of judgements, beliefs, ego, and the multiple I's of personality. During those rare moments in time when we are connected with this essence, it literally floods our being, emanating toward all those around us. They are irresistibly drawn in to that which is truth - the truth of who we are. In these rare moments, we become consciously aware - we come out of our normal state of waking slumber, and look in wonder and awe upon the world. We exude a natural state of enthusiasm in this heightened condition of awareness, for at this point we are beyond the lower frequencies of emotional energy, and have come into a space which allows us to experience wholeness of being in its truest sense.

From this inner space, which is not a place in a physical sense, we can perceive truth. We become aware (recognize) that all "problems" and situations in our lives, and opinions and concepts about ourselves, are self-created; indeed, they are only projections of our mind. Polarity consciousness and our usual linear thinking are temporarily abated, and we can now see both sides of an issue. The pieces of the puzzle, which are the fragments of self, fall together in seconds, so that we can now observe the whole picture. It is as if we get a brief glimpse behind the curtain of our personality. This whole process may last a few minutes, and often only a few seconds, and then suddenly, as if in a twinkling of an eye, we are asleep again, robotically going through the motions of our everyday lives.

Most people experience a deep connection to the Core Self at least once in their lives, such as at the birth of a baby, a wedding, or other deeply moving experience. Some of the shorter moments in life, such as at the observation of a breath taking sunset, when all thoughts about past and future recede into the background and only the beauty of the present moment exists, are the times when we also connect with that inner essence. Such experiences tend to bolster our spirit, giving us a true sense of who we really are, and why we are really here, for we have momentarily broken through the multifarious I, and recaptured a sense of self. To regain a more permanent contact with the Core Self which is our own individuated piece of the divine whole, we must ultimately die to the various I's which have kept us bound in the illusion of separateness. What is needed are techniques which will help us regain contact with the inner self on a more regular basis. The primary method for contacting the Core Self, which involves self observation, is meditation.

During meditation we discover that the concepts and

opinions of the ego are illusory thought forms surrounding the Core Self like layers of an onion. In meditation we have the opportunity to "watch the mind go by." We observe that a myriad of thoughts come and go like phantoms in the night, not one having any real connection with the Core Self. We discover that our thoughts, ideas and beliefs are not truly who we are, but only interpretations of experience, and our concepts about reality. All of these thoughts, ideas, and beliefs have helped to keep us in a constant somnambulistic state. Sometimes only a shock like the loss of a job or a sudden death of a loved one, each of which takes us out of daily routine, will wake us up from our permanent state of sleep.

Most of the time, we don't even realize that we are in this state of waking slumber, and that the majority of a so-called "conscious" day is spent in a state similar to that of hypnosis. Nearly everyone has experienced this situation. How often have you "awakened" after you've missed your exit on the freeway?

We are so lost in this state of unconsciousness that we tend to lose the connection with our Core Self. We thus forget who we are and that we actually have access to the Core Self in every moment.

It is possible to get in contact with the core self quite unexpectedly without any outer cause or stimulus. Anne, a forty-six year old woman described such an experience, "I went home by subway. It was crowded with tired, angry-looking people. The air was stuffy. While absentmindedly regarding the situation, suddenly an idea came to me. How could I be so sure that the situation was really as I perceived it? Was it only my own projection? In the same moment my whole perception changed. It was as if the whole world stopped for a moment. The person named Anne going home from the office disappeared. Suddenly I could see the whole picture and that I was a part of it. Simultaneously I was everything and nothing. Everything was wonderful and unique exactly as it was, including the so called "angry-looking" people. I'm not quite sure how long the experience lasted, I only know it changed my life. Since that day I find myself reminding myself to wake up - to become conscious."

An experience such as the one above, has been described by Maslow as a peak experience. Such experiences can happen at any time, and when they do, they sometimes change the consciousness of the person forever. Most people feel a deep sense of spiritual awakening afterward, not in any religious sense, but in a true openness and caring for those around them. The world suddenly takes on a new perspective, and an unexpected sense of oneness with all that is begins to envelop the person.

The key to the above experience is that Anne was truly awake during her experience - awake in a new way, to the point that later she kept reminding herself to wake up so she could achieve that same sense of being. What was clear was that, to be in such a state, one had to have a heightened sense of awareness. Thus, to live a truly fulfilled life, we have to awaken; we have to become aware.

Peak experiences help to provide further motivation for developing conscious awareness because they show us the truth of who we are and who we are not. Indeed the more consciousness we develop, the easier it becomes to get in contact with the Core Self. Once in contact with the Core Self, we tend to maintain a greater sense of wholeness, and in turn develop confidence in its guidance. It is at this point that the real work begins. We then have the opportunity to lay down our masks, and speak and act from the heart.

Excercise:

The Big Screen

This exercise should be performed in the evening just before retiring. While sitting or lying comfortably, relax your entire body. Close your eyes and take nice long slow deep breaths filling the belly, and slowly exhaling. Now imagine a big screen in your own private movie theater. Begin to review the scenes of the past day. It is not necessary to examine them in a particular order. Just allow the different scenes to appear naturally. Try to recall as many details as possible; for example, thoughts, feelings, conversations, memories, sensory perceptions, and inner comments and judgements which may have passed through your mind about different situations. Don't judge the events or scenes, but observe them from the neutral aspect of the witness self. At the end of the movie turn off the projector, and leave your inner movie theater.

Chapter 2

Rigor Mortis of the Mind

When we come in contact with the Core Self, we see clearly that the true essence of who we are, is not located in the mind. In order to perceive the core self, we must indeed release the mind, which is no easy task, as it is composed of many parts. The mind perceives our thoughts, feelings, and senses, and interprets them under the guise of its many aspects. Some of its aspects include: the intellect, which is our capacity to use logic and reason; the conscious mind, which perceives the various stimuli in our present environment; the unconscious mind, which registers all of our experiences in the nervous system and replays them as needed (and sometimes when not needed), and finally, the ego, which we have created, keeps us identifying with the various I's of the personality. As a child, we create an ego in order to provide ourselves with an identity through which we may express the self. By the time most people reach adulthood, the ego has become overly obsessed and identified with the personality. It has become identified with the personality's various masks and now thinks of itself as "me" or the main "I". The true "me" is now buried in all the confusion. In truth the ego has no center, for it is a product of the mind created by us, but we have long forgotten that it is just that - a product of mind.

The mind is a tool which we use to create the kind of world in which we live. We can use it in a conscious way by being actively involved in the creation of our own reality or, more likely as with most people, we may use it unconsciously, only reacting to life's circumstances.

Most meditators who have developed what many call the

"witness self", are aware of the very mechanical nature of the mind. Like a broken record, the mind will replay old thoughts, images, and emotions which are crystallized and imbedded in both the physical and mental bodies. When certain events occurred in the past and we formed impressions or judgements about them, we set up a pattern which continues to draw similar circumstances to us. The mind then becomes conditioned by the repetition of these self-same circumstances or events, similar to Pavlov's dog which salivated at each ringing of the bell, expecting to receive another meal. The way we think, indeed the very structures we use to approach life, which are conditioned by our parents, teachers, culture and the educational system, are what sets us on the path of this mindless repetition. Similar to old worn out tapes, these old conditioned responses will replay themselves endlessly until we choose to wake up and shine the light of conscious awareness on them. For most of us, it is not always a matter of choice - we are often jolted out of this "rigor mortis of the mind" by the painful effect of a negative reaction to an old outmoded conditioned response pattern.

It seems we blindly keep recreating old patterns in robotic fashion. We generally continue to do so until a pattern is repeated enough times, that we begin to notice the very "obvious," - that there is indeed a pattern, so we may begin to make efforts to change it. One common example in life is a person who marries, becomes dissatisfied, gets divorced, remarries, becomes dissatisfied, gets divorced , remarries, becomes dissatisfied, gets divorced, remarries......then finally steps back and notices (if he or she is lucky) that he has manifested the same type spouse, the same "problems" over and over again. The realization may also come that perhaps the real change needs to happen inside oneself; not in the other person. As we can see from the above, it is understandable how rigid crystallized beliefs and expectations can become a rat trap. A pattern repeated enough times will eventually make itself obvious. Thus it is a comforting thought that crystallized thought forms or beliefs, eventually draw back to us the very experiences we need to have, to destroy them. Such reactivity and blind adherence to old crystallized thought forms permeates all of life.

John Ray, the developer of Body Electronics, contends that all human beings, with very rare exception, are 99% reactive, and that this is due not only to crystallization at a mental level but also at a very physical level as well. (Refer to chapter 5) Anyone familiar with Gurdjief or Ouspensky (or who has maintained a discipline of self-work) is aware of the depth of our reactivity. Most people, when they first hear that we are 99% reactive, totally asleep, and lacking any real conscious awareness, have a strong reaction. "Of course I'm conscious," is a common response, "I make my own decisions. They rarely even consider the conditioning which has most undoubtedly affected these so-called "decisions." After a bit of disciplined self observation however, the obvious sinks in; we are indeed extremely reactive. In addition, it should be noted that whenever we are thinking about what we didn't do yesterday, or what we need to do tomorrow, and are not conscious of the present moment, we are also very much asleep. Thus we are unconscious of the fact that we are always so consumed with the past and future. The mind, with all its various aspects, keeps us totally engrossed in worrying and planning, rationalizing and formulating. We desperately need tools to help us break through these mental habits. Similar to the thorn we can use to take out another thorn, we must also learn to use the mind to get through the mind, to neutralize its unnecessary aspects.

One of the biggest determinants of our conditioning is education. In western society, we are trained in school to define a problem and find a solution. Most of our technical progress is geared along this very line. We are trained to use logic and rationalization to explain reality. Intuition is hardly ever considered. Thus to know something, and not be able to explain why we know it, is considered inadequate. In addition, to respond to our teachers with "I don't know," or "I don't understand," is often taken as a confession of failure. We are expected to find an answer; and it should have a rational-logical format. Constantly we are in a state of "thinking about a solution." Our whole life is lived as if we were continually trying to find a mathematical solution to life's "problems." We are never taught to just be here, now.

How much or how far can we really trust answers delivered by a mind which is conditioned by past circumstances? How fundamental or original can such conditioned thoughts be in regard to creating a new reality? The very structure of the problem solving process itself leads to failure. Robert Fritz, in 'The Path of Least Resistance,' points out that,"the problem leads to action to solve the problem - (which) leads to less intensity of the problem - (which) leads to less action to solve the problem - (which) leads to the problem remaining." In problem solving, we are only taking action to make something go away. If on the other hand we choose to accept life as a challenge rather than a constant problem to be solved, we take the creative tack, for creating is taking action to help something manifest into being - that which we are creating.

It is clear that we have a great creative challenge in the next twenty years - to take the next big step on the path to wholeness, birthing ourselves and reconnecting with the heart of the Core Self. It is a mighty task and we will learn to do it with the help of this wondrous vehicle called the mind.

Exercise:

Mental Circles

After performing The Big Screen, in chapter one a few times, the following exercise will further your efforts in self-observation. Begin by writing down the thoughts and feelings which come to you most often, during the day. Which topics or themes do you seem to dwell on the most? What feelings do they evoke? Notice any recurring patterns and how they affect your daily life. Begin a journal and continue this process on a daily basis. Keep details of the various thoughts, reactions, and emotions which come up around these subjects. Occasionally review your journal and notice the progression of your thoughts, and the changes and shifts in consciousness which may or may not occur.

Chapter 3

Hear No Evil, See No Evil, Speak No Evil

(*Judgement: The Death of Possibilites*)

As we speed along through the challenging Nineties, through to the year 2000 and beyond, the rate at which we must face our past mistakes increases in quantum leaps. We are moving so fast, that as we repeat old patterns or causes we have created in the past as a reaction to certain seed judgements, we are noticing the resulting effects returning to us quicker and quicker. Popular culture refers to this phenomenon as "instant karma." Thus many of us are presently being forced to notice our rigid mental structures as we are pressed to feel instantly the painful effects of our negative reactions brought on by out-moded conditioned response patterns.

Indeed, many of us are being jolted into "semi-consciousness" whether we like it or not, and the more we accept this flow, the less pain and suffering will result. If you are at a point where you are ready to accept whatever tools you can get your hands on to help get you through the labyrinth of mental "stuff" to ease your pain, what you must realize is that to run away or try to squelch your pain is just what will keep it going. You must learn to look at your pain as a pointer to the very causal factor of your suffering. Pain is only the effect of our self-induced "problems." Pain is only a symptom. Thus we must use it as a guide to the very inner depths of being, to whatever issue is really out of synchronization with our Core Self.

The tools we need now are ones which will help us face our

pain head on. We should experience pain fully in order to reveal its underlying message. This in turn enables us to release it - with full knowledge and understanding of whatever it is toward which we have resistance. As most observers of life will tell you, whatever we resist, persists. In facing our pain, we begin to face and release our reactivity, which is totally a result of our unconscious conditioned responses. These responses are a reaction to all of our beliefs piled layer upon layer on top of several seed judgements which made long ago, became crystallized in body and mind, and began to magnetize or attract to us a corresponding outward experience. In other words, whatever beliefs we became identified with long ago, affect our whole perception of reality today, and draw to us actual experiences in everyday life, which in turn act to verify those same beliefs.

In Chapter 2 we discussed Reactivity - indeed how human beings are essentially 99% reactive. Reactivity results from being "preconditioned" by certain ideas or thought forms. Our mind reacts in new situations by instantly seeking out information from past situations which may have seemed similar, so that we may act "appropriately" in the present moment. Unfortunately, all of our past experiences are now
colored by the attitude and mood we were in when they first occurred. Past "similar" situations, and our reactions to them are in turn colored by similar situations before them. We build up layer upon layer of experience, in which each incorporates a certain belief or thought crystal, which in turn stems from a certain judgement. Judgement is at the core of every thought crystal, and surrounding that are all of the experiences magnetized by that initial judgement - each experience in turn giving further false validation to our beliefs about those same judgements.

Thus it can be seen that at a deeper level, the famous biblical quote, "Judge not lest ye be judged," is warning us that ultimately when we judge other people or situations, we are in effect laying judgement back upon ourselves. Therefore, whenever we avoid making judgements, we spare ourselves from more bodily blocks, due to an increased amount of thought crystals. This is not to say we should not discriminate in life, only that we should remain neutral in our thoughts and emotions whenever it becomes necessary to make decisions; in other words, to remain detached from the process, yet still conduct ourselves in a caring way. This is also connected with the biblical insight, "To be in the world but not of it."

Ultimately we can use our judgements or thought crystals as a springboard to search out our resisted truths. Whenever we make a judgement about a situation, a person, or ourselves, behind this judgement there is a resistance to a major truth - to something we don't want to see. We can learn a lot about ourselves by observing the seemingly small judgements we make in our lives. The opinions we form of others are most often a direct reflection of some opinion we are holding about ourselves. Also, if we complain about others, this is a good signal that there is generally something we are dissatisfied with in ourselves. Begin to notice your judgements and opinions about others; they will help to lead you to your innermost feelings and beliefs about yourself.

Finally, we are all familiar with the famous, "Hear no evil, see no evil, speak no evil." This statement, so short yet so profound, serves as wise advice to all of us.

Exercise:

The Judgement Walk

Go for a walk for about an hour (30 minutes minimum.) Direct your attention to the many ways we judge everything which crosses our path and to the labels that we put on things: big tree, old house, beautiful landscape, ugly face, pleasant sound, etc. Notice which adjectives come into your mind as you observe your surroundings. Do not try to suppress these judgements, just be aware of how you label everything. If you get lost with your thoughts, bring yourself back into the present. Also observe what is happening internally on a physical as well as a mental level and how you also judge this with descriptions like tense, relaxed, awake, or tired. Avoid inner conversations; register only what is happening in the moment. After completing the walk, return home, relax and notice how much effort is needed initially to stay in the moment.

If you don't have time or opportunity for a walk, you can do this exercise at home while accomplishing a simple task such as peeling vegetables or washing dishes.

The more often you perform this exercise the more conscious you will become of your judgements and interpretations.

Chapter 4

Creation of Thought Crystals

(How Curiosity Killed the Cat)

Love is the basic source of energy which permeates all of life. In its purest form love encompasses reality as a universal whole, without adding or rejecting anything. Love is accepting, and allows everything to happen without judgement. We perceive this unconditional love only when we are aware of the non-dual nature of reality: when we are aware of the wholeness of life. In this state of awareness, we have the ability to tune in with everything that exists. To the degree that we become haunted by our wants and desires, is the degree to which we find ourselves separated from this state of unconditional love. Our desires gnaw at us; we then become focused on one or two things to the exclusion of all others. This leads to a feeling of lack. We then begin to focus on all the things lacking and thus fall into the consciousness of "not having", for always there seems to be something we don't have: a new car, the ideal partner (relationship), interesting job, and finally the perfect means or method to find happiness. As we attain each goal, it very often doesn't fulfill our original expectations, and tends to satisfy us only for a short while. The beautiful newness is soon spoiled, the ideal relationship loses its ideal quality, the interesting job may become a boring routine, and the perfect technique for happiness leads to a dead end. We become disappointed and frustrated, and then set up the next goal to distract ourselves from our misery. We chase after life, searching for meaning like the rat chasing after the proverbial cheese on the wheel-of-life. A circle of repetition ensues: desire > fulfillment > dissapointment > frustration > new desire. We desperately search for the meaning of life, not realizing that life has no innate meaning. Life is! We are here to experience life, to feel life, to learn from it. We recover a level of source; we contact the Core Self and begin to work from our center, when we realize that it is we who assign meaning to our lives. You will recover a level of source at the point when you realize that meaning in life is what you assign it to be, rather than something you find outside of yourself. For the seeker, this is the end of the line.

To understand how we beome so lost in the labyrinth of mental "garbage", it pays to examine the spiral into thought crystallization. At the beginning of this spiral is curiosity. We first notice a possibility which evokes our interest. This possibility is like a passing whim, not totally robbing our attention. If enough curiosity is aroused, however, our thoughts will begin to circle around it. Soon we are irresistibly drawn into its web. The initial curiosity initiates an inner process which soon flows into the next stage: we then want to have it.

We want to have the objects or qualities that others have, or that we perceive them to have; we begin to want to possess the same money, career satisfaction, wealth, success reputation and love. Our attention then becomes bound by what we don't have.

Be not curious in unnecessary matters: for more things are showed unto thee than men understand.

Apocrypha
Eccliseasticus

Soon the desire becomes a compulsion. At this stage we lose our free choice. We then become blind to the deeper inner calling of Core Self. The initial energy behind these desires and compulsions comes from the drive of the ego, seeking confirmation of itself without true value and without meaning. Identified with the ego, we also begin to feel that all these things we desire will bring us security and the assuredness that we are someone. We thus begin to identify with the objects of our desire. At the final stage of this spiral, the permanent pressure to acquire things then goes hand in hand with resignation and despair. Disappointment and failure build up, making us feel incapable as human beings. Thoughts like "I can't do that", "That's too difficult", "I'll never be able to have that", begin to instill in our consciousness and sink down into the subconscious where these thoughts begin to direct actions and reactions, indeed our very life course. Desires, compulsions, and resignation become self-perpetuating and eventually form a fixed belief system, which in turn attracts experiences confirming the self same belief system.

The limits of our beliefs then determine the limits of our experience. Thus it is when we focus on one particular or limited reaction quite unconsciously in a life situation, with disregard to other possibilities, that the otherwise open wave form of limitless possibilities becomes crystallized into a solid particle or idea of how things are. We then begin to focus on only one "color", out of an otherwise infinite spectrum of possible realities. Thought crystals now act as filters which sort out any areas of reality which disagree with our preconceived ideas or beliefs. The rest of reality then becomes as shadows hidden in the corners of our mind.

On the mental level, thought crystals restrict the flow of awareness, thus limiting our ability to acquire true knowledge. On the emotional level, they block the free flow of feeling, and eventually on the physical level these crystals later manifest as stress, disease, and pain. On the physical level, sensory perception is also affected by thought crystals. The input from our senses is the raw material of our experience, which gets interpreted in a special order and brought into a meaningful context. Our beliefs, which are the content of our mental programs, determine how the sensory raw material is then interpreted and how it takes on meaning. Sensory perception is thus the input which goes into the "computer" hardware or brain, and is interpreted or filtered by our "software," which are the programs and thought crystals stored throughout the body. The "output" is the information which is filtered by our "software" program. How the data is interpreted depends on the capacity and quality of the "software", which is in turn determined by the amount of thought crystals or "mental blocks" we have collected. As long as thought crystals repeatedly spit out the same programs, as do computer chips, true freedom of thought and action remain a virtual impossibility. Life thus becomes a tiring pattern of repetition. The only difference between the life of a rat in a cage and such a life of patterned repetition is the amount of stimuli. How do we escape from such a cage? One very common remedy is offered by positive thinkers. Through affirmations, we are told we can exchange our negative program for positive ones. What most of us do not realize, however, is that by placing a positive charge on top of a negative crystal, there is no guarantee we will be lead out of the prison of unconsciousness. It is equivalent to giving a prisoner a special favor, so that he'll temporarily forget the misery of his position. There is a wonderful German expression which says it aptly, "Es ist wie Schlagsahne auf Scheisse", (It's like putting whipped cream on shit). Crystallized beliefs, whether "positive", or "negative", bind us and keep us dependent on them in different areas of our lives; in our thinking, actions, relationships, and in our communication. It is a miracle that relationships occur at all because there is so little true communication in the world. We do not really talk to each other or share; we talk "at" each other. We actually only list our opinions and concepts about each other. Normal everyday communication is much like watching a newscast: we do not really get the feelings and direct experience of the subjects involved, we get an impersonal account of someone's opinion or concept about what is happening. We tend to do the same thing in daily life; we talk around and about ourselves rather than from the truth of self. When do we really say what we truly think or feel? We wear masks of friendliness, attention and understanding, behind which hide anger, impatience, and boredom. We don't hear each other because our words, thoughts, and feelings are not on the same frequency. Words, voice and body language give contradictory messages. Fixed crystallized opinions about "others" (those who are not me) are like invisible partitions, thus inhibiting the possibility of a true and vital sharing.

Communication on an ego level results only in small talk (thus leaving out any feeling of true commitment or feeling). Most of the time we are enclosed in a thought crystal, busy thinking about a "problem," which totally absorbs the energy we would otherwise use for communication. As a consequence, we don't perceive the other communication partner in his own uniqueness. In observing people who have lived together for a long time, we often notice that they exchange only the information needed for living together without conflict. For example, the type of subjects usually covered are: who will do the shopping, who will do the dishes, who will take little Johnny to the doctor. Each partner can anticipate the reactions of the other and their basic thought patterns. There is no space provided to discover new aspects of the other; no space for the adventure of a real relationship. There is a kind of hidden agreement: "If you don't question my thought crystals, I won't question yours". We are all afraid to talk about our feelings truthfully, as we fear exposing ourselves or damaging our self-image. Our partner might then reject us upon finding out about some of the dark secrets we keep hidden deep inside. Fear also results from our anxiety that we may actually experience something negative about ourselves, which we might not want to face. If it comes out it could destroy our own illusions about ourselves. As a consequence, we prefer to keep to our old familiar ways, where it is safe, and no risk is involved. Thus, thought crystals resulting from long petrified judgements keep our perception of reality in a fixed position and block a full awareness of both ourselves and others.

Each of us lives in a self-created universe with our own set of blinders, reflecting and confirming our own beliefs constantly. The universes we create, each with its own limitations, give us a false sense of security. Our own world feels familiar because "we know", at least we think we know, what will happen next. Everything new and unknown seems frightening because we don't know the results in advance. We might end up lucky and have things go well, or otherwise fall flat on our faces if we attempt to embark on a new journey into the murky unknown. Generally most people end up paying the high price of a frustrating relationship, a boring job, or a life frozen in habits and routine, rather than attempting a new path. To face the full state of our aloneness by following the "beat of our own drummer" is a fearful proposition for most. In our society we appreciate freedom as a high goal that we defend and fight for, but who wants to be really free to accept the full responsibility for self that true freedom entails?

The key to finding the true path to freedom involves the conscious dissolution of our thought crystals, leading to a fuller awareness. With the help of this key we can be set free to explore the infinite space of our Core Self. To dissolve thought crystals, we must first become aware that they exist. We need to observe the particular forms they take within ourselves; to do this, we must note our reactions everytime our "buttons get pushed." The first step to dissolving lies in the awareness of our particular form of resistance.

Resistance is our greatest hindrance on the way to wholeness, and at the same time, ironically, our greatest potential; it is frozen energy which we can set free and use to our advantage. Normally, resistance controls our experience of life, and limits all of our thoughts, feelings and perceptions. Anytime we are very quick in justifying or explaining something, it is a very good sign that deep inside we are strongly resisting something. This resistance is an expression of a lack of confidence or trust in life itself, and its flow of constant change. The true beauty of life lies in its unpredictability. Despite all the assurances we have programmed ourselves with otherwise, we cannot insure ourselves against pain, loss, and disappointment. Life is not static. It is overflowing with possibility, and it is up to us to tap into its natural abundance. The sources of our resistance can be uncovered. The previously condensed frozen energy of resistance can then be utilized for a greater cause. If we cease using our energy in order to deny, to justify, or to pretend, we will extend our life force. Thought crystals can be used as a gateway to freedom. We can learn to seek out and dissolve our crystallized thought forms, while neutralizing their polarities which have kept us in a constant state of unconsciousness. We will then begin to sense the very core or essence of self - indeed, we will return home to the state of witnessing where we existed before the materialization of all our thought crystals.

Exercise:

Objects of Desire

Make a list of your most predominant desires. Observe and write down how you arrived at these desires, and how they now affect your life.

Choose one desire and for fifteen minutes focus on all of your thoughts, feelings, and physical images or reactions concerning this desire. Once you are fully engrossed in this desire, begin to distance yourself from it until you can visualize its shape and form off on the horizon of your mental screen. Watch its image recede into the distance, until it disappears. You can repeat this exercise with all of the desires you have previously listed.

Chapter 5

The Biological Aspects of Thought Crystallization in the Body

We have seen how by continually focusing on one object to the exclusion of all others, the thought form which results becomes crystallized, setting off a whole chain of "conditioned" reactions. This leaves us little choice as to how we respond to life's various challenges. In addition, it has been pointed out how the judgements we make in daily life help to make our beliefs rigid and set us further on the road to unconsciousness. With such an overwhelming state of rigor mortis of the mind, just what is happening in the body? How does the body tie into this state of waking slumber, and how can it aid in bringing us back to a state of conscious awareness?

According to Body Electronics, the two main sources of thought crystallization are contained in Constitutional Man and Natural Man. Constitutional Man is described as the physical body, and its DNA. Essentially, it is the sum total of a person's genetic structure inherited through the parents, grandparents, and ancestors. It is pointed out that by using iridology we can observe in the left eye the qualities inherited from our mother, and in the right eye, those qualities derived from our father. Most inherited weak points show up as a closed lesion in the iris, located in the part of the iris which corresponds to the same organ in the body. For example, one woman had a history of diabetes on her mother's side of the family. She discovered she had a closed lesion located in the pancreas area of the left eye. As diabetes is related to a weakness in the pancreas, which in the case of this disease doesn't provide the appropriate amount of insulin to the body, the closed lesion in the left eye corresponded perfectly with her family life history. Fortunately, this weakness can be controlled by correct diet, and with certain techniques, genetic weakpoints can even be corrected; this is then verified by the changes which occur in the iris when closed lesions actually open up in response to therapy. Thus it can be seen from the description of Constitutional Man (the sum total of our genetic inheritance), that the old Biblical saying "The sins of the fathers will be brought down on the sons," is an actual physical reality. Most weaknesses of the body are a reflection of mind. It seems that whenever our ancestors have erred repeatedly or failed to learn a lesson on a mental level, it has been expressed physically and carried down to us in the form of a corresponding weakness or disease. We naturally tend to magnetize conditions which will benefit our learning, so is it not possible that we might also attract a body which would then enhance certain lessons through its own specific weaknesses?

The other source of crystalline mental structure is described as Natural Man, which is the sum total of each individual's experience in all previous incarnations. It could be described as the soul's private collection of past life lessons, learned and unlearned, which continue to keep each person's reaction patterns in effect. Thus, we may be reacting to conditioned patterns from previous lifetimes. Whether you believe in past lives or not, is of little consequence, as it has been found through several therapeutic techniques that "past life" memories come up in people regardless of their beliefs. These may be only memories connected to the collective unconscious or human morphic field. Whatever your explanation may be, for our purposes what is important is that, in the remembering of these experiences, old crystallized thought forms are transmitted, affecting the present in very profound ways. For example: a woman had found herself in constant debate with her father from about age nine. This affected all her adult relationships with men, as she was conditioned to receiving and giving love through debate. As one can imagine, this did not create an ideal situation for a loving relationship. At one point, she "relived" her last lifetime with her father. They had been brothers in a small dynasty in ancient China. Their father, a small warlord, had set them up in constant competition intellectually, and in martial arts duels to see who was the stronger so that he could determine which son should take over as leader of the dynasty. This process was carried out rather than the normal procedure of letting the oldest son take over. As it turned out, the two brothers ended up killing each other in a martial arts duel. Later, through other past-life regressions, the woman discovered that she had returned in all her subsequent lives as a female, in order to learn the feminine role of compassion, and as a reaction to what she considered the brutal male role. After reliving her lifetime in China, she lost her desire to debate her father. He could no longer "push her old buttons" because, with her new understanding, their old conditioned response pattern was laid bare. She no longer had an attachment to being right every time they got into a discussion and her resistance faded away. What is important in this story is not whether she actually lived this past life or not, but that the story itself provided a strong metaphor for change which did indeed occur in her life.

From the above, we see that there may be some very powerful influences at play on a physical level, as well as soul level, which in turn affects the mind through very ancient conditioning. In addition to various outer influences such as people, language, culture, and education which condition us, there are some inward influences as well, such as the above mentioned past lives. Thus, mental conditioning occurs at many different levels.

The above examples of natural man and constitutional man illustrate how the body provides succinct maps of much of our prior conditioning. In addition, the sensations of the body also provide powerful pointers to our mental programs. It has already been pointed out how pain, when fully and consciously acknowledged, will lead us straight to our crystallized thought forms, for pain is a direct reflection of resistance. The following is a synopsis of an explanation from Body Electronics of how mental resistance affects our awareness, and in turn the physical body: "The natural flow of Cerebral Spinal Fluid is arrested where there is a blockage in the corresponding portion of the electronic body; this occurs whenever a natural law of the human mind is violated. A thought pattern, word pattern, or emotional pattern tempered by resistance of any kind will obstruct or warp the electronic structure of the body. Consciously held thoughts, words and emotions will draw into physical reality the exact physical manifestation of the spiritual prototype which was consciously held in a state of creation. 'Like attracts like.' This is also true of unconscious thoughts. If there is a resistance (on either a conscious or unconscious level), then we will create what we have resisted."

In short, whatever we believe, or think, is just what we will experience, for our experience of reality is a direct reflection of the beliefs that we create. In turn, to whatever extent we resist any life experience we will also become unconscious to the same degree. It is interesting to note that by using a galvanometer (which registers galvanic skin response) to register levels of resistance, it has been found that males register 12,500 ohms of resistance and females 5,000 ohms, because of the difference between the characteristics of the male and female physical structures. If the body were to hit 0 degrees resistance, it would then become a superconductor, and we would then hit the time - space continuum, or "mental level" where all knowledge is absorbed unhindered by blocks or affected by stored thought crystals. Total awareness is then possible, as there would no longer be blocks hindering consciousness. It is interesting to note that the very nature of a superconductor is such that it has no electrical energy loss, as energy loss is due to moving electrons colliding with imperfections in a crystal lattice or structure; this is much like knowledge or truth colliding with the thought crystals or judgements stored in our own body/mind structure, which then acts as a filter to that same knowledge or truth. From the above, we can see men may have a more difficult time than women releasing blocks as resistance is built in to a greater degree; there are more filters due to the very density of male physical structure.

In addition to physical and mental resistance, the state of emotion we are in when we are confronted with any situation, will also determine our level of awareness at that time. Resistance is the key issue, though, which will keep conscious or unconscious thoughts in a constant state of creation, and result in a corresponding reduction in physical life energy. Mental resistance first manifests in the etheric or energy body also known as the bioplasmic body. The blockage can then carry down to a corresponding

area of the physical body depending on which emotion or issue is involved. In addition, thought crystallization occurs as a result of thoughts or emotions which get suppressed, and the crystals themselves lodge in the same body part which does the suppressing. The physical body thus becomes the repository of our thought forms and emotions, which in turn often cause disease. It behooves us then to work on ridding ourselves of outmoded patterns and to begin thinking about developing conscious awareness.

Discovering Body Crystals

List all of the major illnesses and accidents which have occurred in your life. Think back to the circumstances which were happening in your life at the time they occurred. Can you see any connection between each accident or illness and your emotional state and thought patterns at that time? What were you preoccupied with then? What were your personal relationships like? Have these patterns occurred repeatedly in your life? Are you suffering from a chronic illness? Again note the time and circumstances of its first occurrence, and its secondary benefits to you now. To help release these patterns, use the exercise in chapter 8.

Chapter 6

Feelings Express Truth Clearer than Words

The most successful prophets, artists, inventors, and businessmen are those who are tuned into their feelings. In school we are taught how to think, to use reason and logic, which are excellent tools for solving mathematical type problems; yet we are rarely taught in public schools how to develop our intuitive abilities or to trust our feelings. As a result, people who succeed in creative endeavors are generally those who are either self-taught or innately gifted. The public is slowly catching on, though. This can be seen through the many publications which explain how to succeed in business by developing intuition.

Intuition is in part the ability to sense the feeling behind symbols and, as in the case of an artist, to be able to translate feelings into symbols that will also arouse similar feelings in others. An artist uses color and form to portray feelings. A writer uses words, carefully choosing his adjectives to arouse certain emotions in the reader. In addition, the prophet or artist tunes into the collective unconscious, to express what the masses are feeling before it actually manifests in physical form. They are "ahead of the pack" simply because they can feel the tone of the collective mental landscape and express it for, as we all know, form follows thought.

The connection between intuition and feeling can also be seen when observing the seven main energy centers in the body, also known as Chakras. The heart chakra is the middle energy center, with three above and three below it. The second chakra located four finger widths below the navel, also called the chi or ki center in martial arts, is known to be the center of our feelings. This is expressed in everyday phrases such as "I have a gut feeling," or "I can't stomach another ...," etc; all alluding to the energy center of our feelings.

The corresponding energy center above the heart which is known as the sixth chakra, and sometimes the third eye, is our center of intuition. It is here that we tune into symbols, which may be words or pictures, on the mental level. We then integrate this information, with the feelings we have received from the ki center, if we are open in these two chakras.

Neither feelings nor intuition derive from a logical, rational process, yet feelings rather than logical rational decisions, as some people might think, are our prime motivation for action. Indeed our prime motivation for action is either to feel something or to avoid feeling something. People whose purpose is to feel, create; those whose purpose is to avoid feelings, think.

We have already examined how people who feel, create. Most of us have experience in rationalization and logic. It would also pay to examine our actual styles of thinking to see just how we so conveniently avoid feeling.

There are many different styles of thinking. Two of the basics are literal and figurative. When you have a literal and a figurative thinker involved in a conversation, the two will often be at odds with each other misinterpreting meaning, and projecting each one's ideas on the other's words. In essence, words have different meanings for different people. The figurative thinker tends more towards symbols. He uses metaphors to express himself, often exaggerating with words to make a point. The literal person often misunderstands figurative speech, as he tends to stick to the precise meaning of words, and often even misses the pun in jokes. There are also those who combine both of these mental traits, using them to suit each situation. A good example is a person who uses figurative speech to describe another in a negative way - yet becomes quite literal when it comes to describing his own "rightness." He becomes downright prosaic, often demanding exact literal retorts from his opponent, contrary to his own original figurative speech. In synopsis, we tend to use any thinking pattern which will suit our needs in the moment. Our reactions to life's situations are mostly unconscious, thus we quickly "draw from the pot," whichever thinking mode best offers the quickest response in any given situation. We talk and rationalize until we are blue in the face, often missing the real issues which are involved, totally missing our own deeper feelings and those of others.

As our ego connects with our deeply rooted survival instincts, in its own quest for survival, we become addicted to being right. When we do this, we shut out our sensitivity to other people's feelings. We also often receive another's insensitivity as an attack, and unconsciously respond at their level of (Ego) thinking. Talking is an offshoot of the thinking process, thus it is truly rare that we ever really communicate with words. We tend to talk "at" one another not only on the job, but also in normal social situations. The fact that we "make" conversation is an apt description in itself. True communication really comes through our facial expressions, our eyes, our body language, and the sound of our voice, in response to another. An example is the person who says with a tight clenched jaw, how "wonderful" he's feeling today. From this illustration we can see how it is, that the body really tells the truth.

It is interesting to note how many artists have expressive body language, as they tend to communicate outwardly the same feelings they express in their art. Indeed we could even change a previous statement to read: People whose purpose is to create, feel, and people whose purpose is to think, avoid feelings.

From all of the above examples, we can see that words are not particularly effective for communicating experiential clarity. In fact, life becomes complicated to the degree that symbols (words) are substituted for feelings. Feelings are primary on a basic energetic level.

It has been noted that people in the same room who cannot or do not talk, such as in a waiting room, eventually will feel the same, or resonate at the same level. Just as water naturally finds its own level, energy also naturally finds its own balance. We can see how powerfully the vibratory level of feelings or emotions of persons within our vicinity, can affect our own feelings, because feelings are so much more powerful than words.

Feelings are alive in the moment; they speak the truth of who we are now. To note our true feelings in any moment is to be conscious and fully aware in that moment. Words can only be used to create a description of a real feeling or object. They have no reality in and of themselves. We create an illusory world with words. In turn, these words may provoke certain emotional reactions, leading us into more illusion. We can then lose our feel of the present moment and become lost in the past or future, or in some other "imaginary reality."

It is important to note at this point the essential difference between feelings and emotions. To feel is to be aware or conscious of an inward impression, state of mind, or physical condition. An emotion can be thought of as a very intense feeling, which often is expressed outwardly. As mentioned above, emotions are often provoked by words. We call forth emotions in ourselves when we dwell on the past or unnecessarily worry about the future. At other times, emotions are provoked when we react to another person through our past conditioning. A typical example is a person in a new relationship who reacts negatively to something his partner says in total innocence, but which seems reminiscent of something negative from a past relationship. When we react emotionally, we are generally expressing feelings which relate to past events, and like most of our thinking processes, these reactions are also almost all unconscious.

We have seen how important it is to be in touch with our feelings in order to become more conscious in the present moment. In addition, we have observed how, when we are in

48

a thinking mode, we are generally unaware of our true feelings. What must also be considered is how emotions tend to dominate our conscious state. Because emotions are so powerful, most of them, like the thinking mode, tend to put us in an illusory state.

Body Electronics uses a chart of the seven main emotions to illustrate how powerfully certain emotions will keep us in a somnambulistic state. To understand further, we must refer to the following chart:

ENDOCRINE GLAND	LEVEL OF EMOTION	DEGREE OF MEMORY
1) Pineal	ENTHUSIASM	Impartial Memory (can now see other 'both' sides of view)
2) Pituitary	PAIN	Capstone to Memory (Kundalini level)
3) Thyroid/ Parathyroid	ANGER	Specific Memory (one-sided)
4) Thymus	FEAR	vacilates specific memory between general memory
5) Pancreas/ Adrenals	GRIEF	General Memory (victim level)
6) Spleen	APATHY	No Memory (cannot remember)
7) Gonad	UNCON-SCIOUSNESS	No Memory (cannot remember)

At first glance when viewing the above chart, we notice a dividing line through fear. When we are absorbed by any of the emotions below the fear level, and sometimes at the fear level itself, we feel much like a victim of circumstance. We feel as though we are at the mercy of those around us and that we have little or no control in our lives. When we are consumed by these dense lower vibratory emotions, it is virtually impossible to feel as if we have any control over determining cause in our lives. This is in contrast to a fully realized person who makes his own decisions and chooses his own goals, effectively steering his own course, and being the true creator of cause in his life. Such a creator of cause lives not in an artificially created enthusiasm, which acts as a cover for true feelings, but in a natural state of enthusiasm emanating from the Core Self. The opposite is thus the victim level, where one would feel the victim of circumstance; he would feel very much influenced by his environment.

A recognizable example, which illustrates the progression through the different levels illustrated on the chart, is the experience of emotional healing after the unexpected death of a loved one. Often a person may experience a mild form of shock, or may even go unconscious or become numb (apathy) when the death is first announced. Soon at the grief level, we pour out our woes, "How could this happen to me?" we ask. We feel the victim of circumstance, as we feel at the effect of the situation. Soon we reach the fear level, where we begin to face reality, yet from a very one-sided vantage point. "Just how will we survive without them?" is the common feeling. However, we have finally reached the dividing line between cause and effect. From this point, we can begin to move beyond the survival level mentality of effect.

After some time, anger will arise: anger at the dead person for leaving us. We are beginning to perceive cause, but still from a one sided viewpoint. Our memory is specific to our experience, as another's viewpoint (the dead person's) is not considered. Eventually we face the real pain of loss and, if we are willing to truly experience our pain fully, to express it, and let it go, we finally move up to the level of enthusiasm. Pain is the capstone to memory, where we begin to see and understand both sides of an issue. This is the level where we find real movement. Pain is at the kundalini level, which moves the energy and where even physical regeneration can occur. When we accept our pain with enthusiasm for all that life has brought us, and accept our suffering as a path, a guide post to the lessons we need to learn, we can finally progress to the level of impartial memory, where we can see both sides of any situation. We can then accept both life and death. At this point, we begin to feel really alive. The experience of death has finally given us a true appreciation of life.

Love and enthusiasm will transmute through the various levels of emotion. Therefore it is extremely important to experience all of our feelings fully with enthusiasm, even the most negative or painful. To feel emotions such as grief or pain with enthusiasm may seem contradictory, however it is not meant that we should be masochistic or dwell on these like a martyr, only that we should experience them completely with a full bodied conscious attention, so that they can finally be transmuted. All feelings must be acknowledged. Nothing should be suppressed or buried, saved for a rainy day to pop up later when we least need it. Another important point to remember is, when we move up from one level to another, that we don't get stuck short of enthusiasm. One common phenomenon is the depressed person who with the help of therapy moves higher up the emotional chain to a level of anger, where he begins to express his long buried feelings. He begins to feel very good expressing anger, as it is a much higher vibratory frequency than grief or apathy, and he soon gets stuck in a merry-go-round of emotional acting out. Anger is the step just before we face our real pain. We must take real courage at this point. We must remind ourselves that by accepting our pain lovingly and willingly it will be transmuted quickly. It is not necessary or even desirable to wallow in the pain, it is only important that we don't resist it. We must gather up our resources of love and enthusiasm and transmute through the final layer of pain so that we can finally access a true level of enthusiasm, where the realm of opposites disappears.

At this point it becomes possible to encompass the original seed judgement, and holographically experience all memories connected with one polarity. When we are in a true state of enthusiasm, we can then experience the opposite duality, which makes it possible to bring both polarities together and dissolve them.

Finally we have transmuted the realm of opposites, reaching a state of neutrality. With duality no longer controlling us, we regain our ability to choose, to truly make our own decisions and become the cause in our life. No longer are we the victim of circumstances, seemingly at the effect of others. We then begin to create our own lives, choosing love and enthusiasm to light our way.

Think enthusiastically about everything; but especially about your job. If you do, you'll put a touch of glory in your life. If you love your job with enthusiasm, you'll shake it to pieces. You'll love it into greatness; you'll upgrade it, you'll fill it with prestige and power.

Norman Vincent Peale

Exercise:

Experiencing Enthusiasm

Recall a situation when you have been very angry. Focus intently on the feeling evoked by the situation, rather that the actual context. Once you have re-activated the feeling of anger, begin to expand it. Feel it move throughout your entire body and expand outward in all directions. Once you feel the outer limit of its expansion, begin to contract the anger back inside of yourself. You may use your breath with this exercise, expanding as you exhale, contracting as you inhale. Repeat the expansion and contraction several times, and then choose a different situation of feeling to work with, when you have been consumed by enthusiasm. Experience the expansion and contraction of enthusiasm. You can use this exercise with other feelings, or with some of the thoughts you observed while keeping the journal described in the Mental Circles exercise.

Chapter 7

The World of Polarities

As long as we have lived on the earth and existed in a physical form, human beings have been engrossed in the realm of opposites. Polarity seems inherent in everything. In truth we are really one. However, because we are unconscious of that fact, and see ourselves as dual, we tend to recreate more of that same duality. Fortunately, the result is that through the friction and opposition of these polar opposites, we are ultimately made to understand our unity.

While living in matter, our whole perception of reality is based on making comparisons and observing opposites. We understand our internal world and the surrounding environment by measuring it in relation to something else: light and dark, hot and cold, life and death. Without these comparisons, it would be difficult to perceive reality. We would not even be able to discern the difference between objects, as we would observe one large blur, much like a newborn infant; shape or form itself is recognized by comparing it to something which it is not. For example, we recognize a chair only by comparing it to everything that is NOT a chair. In our normal everyday life we are totally dependent on our sensory perception. Even the basic philosophy of mainstream science stipulates that what we cannot touch, smell, or measure in a physical sense is not real. It is only due to recent developments in quantum physics that scientists are now considering alternative realities.

We experience polarity in ourselves, and in the world around us. It appears in the rhythms of nature: day and night, fall and spring, winter and summer, and the ebb and flow of the tides. In our bodies, opposites affect the very life process:

heating and cooling, inhaling and exhaling, anabolizing and catabolizing, digestion and excretion. Our minds are especially affected by polarities: right and wrong, good and bad, important and unimportant. Even communication itself depends on descriptions based on opposites, otherwise there would be no basis for comparison.

Every pole is totally dependent on its opposite, as it cannot exist without its other half. They both have a shared basis, a point as it may, where they come together. The perception of polar opposites is dependent on our existence in time and space. It is nearly impossible for us to perceive things at the same time, as time in our dimension puts things in a certain order, everything happening one after another, on a linear basis. Once we transcend this time limitation, we then open up to the possibility of experiencing the union of opposites.

The effects of polarity are so natural on our everyday lives, so all encompassing, that we rarely think about it or question whether it is the only way things are. We rarely think about the power which brings opposites into existence.

The age old wisdom of Hermetic science sheds much light on the realm of opposites. The real roots of this knowledge are unknown, although the fact that it appeared in Egypt under the tenets of Thorus the God of Wisdom, prior to its introduction to Greece, is generally accepted. The first three laws of Hermes Trismegistrus, the Greek God of Wisdom, pertain to the absolute, for they are non-dual in nature. The first law, "All is Mind", refers to a universal mind (the mind of God) manifested on an infinite scale of vibration, each producing the different elements of the universe. The second, is the law of Correspondence, "As above, so below...As it is below, so it is above," and the third, the law of Vibration, states that "Everything moves, that all is vibration." The last four laws of Hermetic science describe the conditions which govern our lives, for they also describe the circumstances under which life in matter operates: The fourth law states "Everything is double; everything has two poles; each has its opposite." The fifth, sixth, and seventh laws are the laws of rhythm, (up and down, forward and backward); the law of cause and effect; and finally the law of gender (male and female). Indeed, out of seven main laws in Hermetic science, the last four deal specifically with polarity. The first three laws are considered to describe reality, whereas the last four laws describe an illusory state, that of duality, which we must ultimately transcend in order to become whole or unified. Duality should never be considered a negative or "bad" state as it affords us the circumstances which are a necessary opportunity for choice and learning. When we truly understand this concept, we will begin to see through the illusion of separation. We will then be able to see others in us, and ourselves in others.

Although we recognize most of these principles intellectually, we must realize that duality affects us on a very basic level, and is most often very tricky to deal with. Everything we become attached to or identify with has its polar opposite, which is generally hidden to ourselves and thus refered to as a shadow. We are just as controlled by the "shadow", as the actual side of the polarity we are "consciously" identified with, if not more so. Before we can reach a state of unity, we must become conscious of the polarities with which we are identified, and in addition root out their opposites or shadow aspects. We must then bring each of the polarized opposites together and neutralize them to attain real freedom.

An excellent example of bringing two polarized opposites together can be illustrated on a broad scale by examining recent history. For years Marxist and Capitalist doctrines clashed. Each one continually resisted the other, in turn feeding each other with more energy to keep the clash going. Remember, "Whatever you resist, persists?" The cold war continued for many years until each side undid itself of its own accord. In the West, people focused too much on the almighty dollar. They gave up their personal power to greed, and destroyed most of the economy in the process. In the East, people yielded their personal power to the governments. People gave up their autonomy in exchange for having the government take care of the entire distribution system for them: food, clothes, and all the basic necessities. The total lack of incentive inherent in this system, due to a giving up of responsibility for self, led to its ultimate downfall. As of this writing much of the West is still teetering on the brink of financial downfall.

Both of these seemingly separate ideologies - Marxism and Capitalism, are really two sides of the same coin. One focused more on taking care of the group as a whole, while the other fostered the development of the individual. Both ideologies provide valid insights, and if put in balance as a whole by taking the best of both, together they could provide a myriad of possibilities for economic success. The key point here is that these two ideologies are only mental structures. They are ideas in our minds, of how things should be. We have shown very concretely that neither is necessarily more valid than the other. The lack of consciousness in the people who supported each of these ideologies led to their ultimate downfall, not the ideological structures themselves. We can see this same lack of consciousness exhibited in the "holy" wars of the old Christian crusaders, and the so- called "holy" war of Saddam Hussein. Any rational person realizes there is no such thing as a "holy" war. Only someone so lost and identified with his judgements and beliefs, that he had forgotten who he really was, could even conceive of a "holy" war.

All of these mental attachments to "my side being the right side," whether it be related to religion, politics, or even more personal issues, all stem from a very old, very ingrained survival skill which unfortunately usually gets the best of us. In primeval times, our minds had to think up quick responses to the many dangerous scenarios which constantly plagued our days. We needed to be "right" quickly to save our skin. If a dangerous animal crossed our path, if a hoard of bandits moved in on our territory, we needed to have a ready answer; we needed to be right as to how to respond NOW. There was no time for rationalization and logic. Instincts were more important because there was no debate between the right or wrong answer. There was only one answer - the right one.

As we can see, in the old days it was very appropriate to be right. Unfortunately in today's world, this trait has become almost second nature. The personality has now attached itself to this need to be right and in the process we make all others (our polar opposites) wrong. Regretably this becomes a bad habit. The resulting effect is that the mind endlessly manufactures wrongness in others, therefore placing blame for the so-called wrong outside of ourselves. Thus, we can see that much of the polarization of the mind is artificial.

This pattern tends to come up a lot when we are unhappy with ourselves. We persistently blame others in our perpetual state of unconsciouness, and react to them in defense when often it is not really due. In addition, when we make the other person wrong, in their own unconscious state, they tend to automatically react, putting us in turn, in the wrong. This merry-go-round of unconscious reacting goes on and on. The only way to stop this process is to become conscious.

Friction is inherent in duality, and the friction gives the illusion of two opposing sides bent upon self-extermination. In actuality, the seeming opposites are self-completing, creating one unique whole. Thus when two opposites come together a sacred trinity is formed, such as when a man and woman come together and create a child. Even religion and science, which today still seem to be such opposing forces, are described by Teilhard de Chardin as being "the two conjugated forces or faces of one and the same complete act of knowledge." Rather than perceiving this sacred union of opposites, normally we only see one side of an issue, and cut off its polar opposite. The challenge then begins, and the resulting "problems" then ensue. This is the beginning of the struggle. The natural flow of open possibilities now becomes interrupted.

On the personal level, there is separation between subject and object. We experience an "I" which feels separate from "the world." To the same degree that we perceive the world to be something separated from ourselves, it becomes similarly difficult to note any of the related qualities in that world. The "Outer World" is thus something threatening, and as a result we resist it and fight it.

The pattern of resistance is based on our identification with our ideas about ourselves, our self image, including their polar opposites, of which we are normally unaware: if someone is deeply attached to becoming a "successful" person, he will tend to shun all people he considers unsuccessful, and avoid contact with them, as they mirror his own unsuccessful element. Thus a person who rarely succeeds, will in turn tend to dislike "successful" people and avoid them. There are a variety of ways that this resistance manifests: envy, jealousy, and rationalizations for one's own conduct. Often there may even be an attempt to "lash out" at the other person who mirrors your polar opposite. Most people with a little self observation will notice this pattern in themselves and others.

When we identify with one thought or idea, its polar opposite disappears behind the veils of the subconscious. Although it is now passively hidden in the shadows, this polar opposite remains fully alive, affecting our life in its own subtle way. It actually refuels its dual aspect, that with which we have become identified, with even more energy. One day it may even reappear at the surface of consciousness and polarize an otherwise well built up self-concept. Such an example is the person who does a total about face, quickly converting to a new religion, or ideology in a very unconscious way.

The only way to stop this process, to finally bring this pattern to completion, is to become conscious. It is only by becoming conscious that we can finally see through the illusion of opposites. The illusion itself is rooted in the senses, and will persist as long as the senses persist.

In order to become whole, it is necessary to deal with polarity in a conscious and honest way. Blaming others only reinforces opposites. When we choose to really face the shadowed aspects of reality, the very shadows within ourselves, we can then dissolve the power of unconscious patterns over us, and even neutralize these polarized aspects and transcend them.

*The realm of Opposites is not hard to find,
in fact it seems to be all there is. The
realm of Absolutes does not exist until you
consciously create it. It is thus a narrow
path rarely even noticed, in fact, not there
until you create it.*

Unknown

Exercise:

Changing Identities

Recall a situation where you have been in a heated conflict or argument with someone. Review all of the thoughts and feelings evoked by the situation. See your "opponent" very clearly in front of you. Now transport yourself into his or her shoes and begin to think his thoughts, to feel his feelings and reactions and note his perception of you. Really see yourself from the other's viewpoint. Do this exercise with all the intensity you can muster. Really feel his feeling, really think his thoughts. Now go back to your own position. How do you feel? What has changed? Notice any shifts in your consciousness.

Chapter Eight

Attachment: The Fun of Being an Earth Addict

There was a story told in ancient times of a group of gods who got together to assess the state of life on earth. As the group closely observed the antics of the people and animals on earth, one of them commented on the great difficulty humans have in attempting to transcend the great pull of matter. She remarked that although there was a great deal of misery and pain to prompt people to further growth, the pleasures and addictions of earth life were too great a pull for most to "live on the earth, but not be of it." Many of the gods murmured agreement, and one also mentioned that so great was the pull and attraction to matter, that indeed it would also be a formidable challenge for any one of them to attempt to take on an earthly body and still remain conscious. One of the gods disagreed. "We have evolved too far," he said, "to get caught up in the attraction to earthly life. To prove it I'll take on a body for six months; to make it even more difficult I'll take on the body of an animal, and I'll return to you at the end of that time."

The other gods were astounded by his challenge, but true to his word he descended to earth and entered the body of a little piglet. At first the god felt awkward to be so restrained in the tight feeling of matter, but soon he became absorbed in the pleasure of sucking his mother's warm teats. He played in the mud with the other little piglets. He grunted and snorted, soon very thoroughly enjoying the pleasure of being a pig. His body grew quickly as he happily stuffed himself with the pig slop the farmer provided, and in no time at all he also became quite a stud.

The gods watched in awe, observing the behavior of their

companion. "He's truly lost in matter," said one. "He may never get out," said another. As the six months drew to a close, a few of the gods went to earth to prod the young pig and remind him of who he truly was. The pig ignored them and happily grunted away eating his slop. No form of prodding or pleas from the other gods worked. In desperation, they finally decided to slay the pig in order to release the god. When they did so, they were shocked to see their friend still groveling on the ground. It took him a long time to recuperate before he really remembered who he was.

As we can see from the story, the god had become an earth addict very much like ourselves. We are all addicts in one form or another: not necessarily drug, food, or alcohol addicts in the usual sense, but we are addicted to the things we become most identified with or attached to. Our needs and wants also lead us into addiction, such as the need for verification that we actually exist. In order not to face the emptiness or vacuum which occasionally looms over us, the void of meaning as it were, we search for things to grasp at, such as people, things or beliefs. We attach ourselves to life in order to avoid the thought of our inevitable death. We become attached to our family and friends because we fear being alone. We attach ourselves to our thoughts because we think they will solve our "problems." We remain attached to our past because it gives the ego a story to identify with. Ultimately we cling to our habits so that we may easily avoid making new choices, for it is far easier to leave our blinders on and follow our old patterns, than to see life "as through the eyes of a child."

Attachment starts at the very beginning of life on earth. As we bond to our mothers, we are at the same time bonding to physical matter itself. The body becomes our sole vehicle for expression in the world, and we thus begin to identify with it as an integral part of who we are. We become totally dependent on its functions for survival, and in turn become bound to it until our physical death. When the body ceases functioning in any way, our freedom of action becomes restricted. For example when we are tired or have a headache, all the levels of being become affected. We can no longer concentrate, or our feelings become blocked. We also identify with a certain image of our body. This image has a strong influence on our actual physical structure. The body image we produce in our mind projects through to the outer world, and in turn affects not only the development of our body, but also influences the way people react to us. Almost everyone has experienced the following situation: On a really good day while looking in the mirror first thing in the morning, you perceive yourself as attractive, and you accept yourself accordingly. This positive image then emanates and gets reflected to you by those you meet during the day, in the form of compliments or friendlier interactions.

In actuality, our body is only one aspect of our being. If we identify too much with its form or its abilities, we become dependent. People who are very concerned about the body and identify with it (such as athletes, dancers, and actors), are especially dependent on its state of health for survival. They tend to identify totally with their physical abilities. If this identity is disturbed by an accident or disease, it may lead to a breakdown.

Being attached to fixed body images, whether positive or negative, reduces the possibility for healing or "wholing" to take place. The way we deal with illness or disease illustrates this. On a superficial level someone may seek a healing and ask for it, but on a deeper level he may really want to keep the disease because of its secondary benefits. For example, by getting sick you then have an excuse to take the needed rest which you have denied yourself for so long. Illness is also a good way to get attention which you would otherwise not receive. For children, it is often the only opportunity they may have to get their busy parents to spend personal time with them at home.

Disease is neither good nor bad. It simply provides us with an opportunity to grow and learn, and to explore deeper levels of our being. In order to learn from disease, we need to be able to step back from it - to see it from a new perspective. This distance helps us to experience new aspects of ourselves which we may not have previously encountered. The following is one example:

Margaret, a very strong woman who is also very successful in her career, reported: "After an accident, I had to spend several weeks in the hospital and could not move. For the first time in my life I was weak and dependent on others. It was a totally new experience for me to accept help from other persons. I felt that others helped me not out of a sense of duty, but actually out of the joy of giving. It made it a real pleasure to receive. As I had always played the strong woman, I had never really given people the opportunity to do something for me. Due to the accident, I learned to accept both my weaknesses and my strengths, and discovered the joy of receiving."

Margaret learned a lot from her experience and didn't view it in a negative way. Any time we give up something we have previously been attached to (as in Margaret's case, her prior regard for strength), it is a good signal that something is opening in us. We now have an expanded space in which to develop a new aspect of ourselves; we can then move on to the next stage of our development. Our consciousness also expands because it is no longer bound within the framework of the previous identification. When we release old patterns, we also often experience an actual physical reaction, for example: mild endothermic and exothermic reactions often occur when releasing very large blocks in consciousness. We can also breathe and relax more easily after relaxing old patterns. In everyday life, we have great difficulties in releasing our patterns because we are generally totally identified with the situation at hand and not able mentally to step outside and view things objectively.

Habit plays a large role in maintaining this form of identification or attachment because habits lead naturally to a state of unconsciousness. We do things as we do them because we have, "always done it like that." We have been trained as children to develop good habits, and thus don't often question whether they make any sense. Habits are not necessarily bad either, as long as we use them consciously. When they dominate us, and we can no longer make spontaneous decisions, often the habits effectively cut us off from direct experience of life. They can become a compulsion and thus "imprison" us in the "power of habit," as an old German saying goes. For example: when we always drive the same way to work, we deprive ourselves of the opportunity to experience something new. Upon giving up habits to which we have long been attached, life can again become an adventure. It can give you a deep feeling of freedom when you change your day completely, and do everything in a fresh new way. We may begin with something as simple as tying your left shoe first instead of your right, just to stimulate conscious action. In the teaching of the Sufi's, giving up old habits and patterns is the first step on the path to freedom, as habits are also deeply connected to the self image. We have a lot of self concepts as to who, what, and how we should be. Identification with these images is very deep. When we feel uncertain, we hang on to these images; when the old ones no longer provide security, we then create new ones. Normally we present only our positive self images to the world and attempt to conceal the negative ones. Despite tremendous effort to keep these images afloat, there is no real foundation for them. We cling to these illusions of self, so that we will not have to face ourselves directly in all our aspects.

When other people criticize us or challenge our self image, this also causes great fear. As children, we learned behaviour patterns which would guarantee love and acknowledgement. We learned to suppress "inappropriate" behavior because we were criticized or rejected for showing negative emotions or acting out our feelings. As adults, we have maintained behavior patterns which continue to elicit approval. We focus on positive qualities which we feel will help us to be more greatly accepted: to be good, honest, helpful, friendly, patient, etc. These can only be maintained by suppressing the so called "negative" qualities and feelings such as anger, jealousy, and dishonesty.

A lot of energy is needed to continue this deception of ourselves and others. By investing all our energy in this game, we lose contact with our inner feelings. To develop inner strength, we have to cease identifying with certain self images which we favor over others, and begin perceiving all the various aspects of ourselves. We can run away from ourselves our whole life, or take the risk to face the truth of ourselves by embracing all of our various I's, the "good" and the very "bad." In the beginning, it may seem scary or difficult; however, if we persevere and observe ourselves without judgement, we will then discover our deepest feelings and abilities.

We must remind ourselves that our bodies and identities are merely steps on a journey through infinite dimensions of being, providing us with an opportunity to try on various experiences and to learn. Life on earth in this space-time dimension can lead us into addictive behavior because there are certain experiences which we will want to have again and again. This is not to say we should not enjoy these experiences, it is only to say we should not become attached to them. The more we release these attachments, the more our consciousness will expand and open to even greater dimensions. It is possible to love things, experiences, and people without being overly attached to them, without becoming dependent. When we finally free ourselves of our earthly addictions, we will enable ourselves to experience the truth of unconditional love. We will then be able to be "In the world, but not of it."

Exercise:

Releasing Attachment

Recall a situation when you have been in a heated conflict or argument with someone. Review all of the thoughts and feelings evoked by the situation. See your "opponent" very clearly in front of you. Now transport yourself into his or her shoes and begin to think his thoughts, to feel his feelings and reactions and note his perception of you. Really see yourself from the other's viewpoint. Do this exercise with all the intensity you can muster. Really feel his feeling, really think his thoughts. Now go back to your own position. How do you feel? What has changed? Notice any shifts in your consciousness.

Chapter Nine

The Challenge of Being in the Present Moment

To be in the moment is to be truly alive and awake in the present: to be totally conscious. By contrast, whenever our mind is caught by a thought which then enters our brain and touches on any issue relating to either the past or future, we fall quickly into sleep, and are soon out of touch with our Core Self. We are constantly consumed by a mental museum of old thoughts, beliefs and judgements. In addition, our patterned web of fleeting thoughts many times evokes emotions which tend to lead us even further away from the present moment. For example, we may be having a perfectly wonderful day, when someone happens to remind us of an unpleasant experience which may have happened days before. Soon we are mentally re-experiencing that earlier episode, ruminating about an event which evokes negative emotions. We then carry those emotions into the present moment, ruining what previously had been a decidedly pleasant day. We are constantly overwhelmed with very similar circumstances. Our thoughts and emotions from previous events play on our minds and keep us continually distracted from being in a true present. We seem to keep a permanently running, pre-recorded tape in our heads spitting out repetitiive thoughts such as, "What do I have to do next?", or "What does he think of me?", "Did I finish what I was supposed to do yesterday?" All of these take us further and further from the present moment.

The beginning of self work is thus a constant challenge. Initially, it takes a lot of discipline and strong desire to fuel any real movement on the path to conscious awareness; ironically, at the same time we must balance our strong desire to become conscious, in effect neutralize it, so we do not become overly attached to the goal. An attachment to becoming an "aware person", can soon be absorbed by the ego and in itself lead us astray.

Many great thinkers have recognized the importance of stepping outside the sequential effect of time, to discover the eternal moment. Aldous Huxley, in his discussion of Perennial Philosophy, pointed out that, "the present moment is the only operative through which the soul can pass out of time into eternity, through which grace can pass out of eternity into the soul, and through which charity can pass from one soul in time to another soul in time." It is true that, to have any kind of real communication or sharing with others, we must be in the present moment with them. Most often, as has been previously mentioned, we usually talk "at" someone if we are mentally in the past or future. From Huxley's quote, we can also see that the present moment affords us the only opportunity to contact the divine. If we are always working "to get there," the result will always be in the tomorrow, thus never quite reaching our goal. We can only experience eternity NOW; we can only accept the grace of the absolute NOW. This constant focus we place on the concept of time, on the importance of past and future, is our constant undoing. The great spiritual master Eckhart stated that, "Time is the greatest obstacle between man and God." He stressed that temporalities, temporal affections, and the "very taint and smell of time ," were all further obstacles to God. Many other great masters from all the different religious traditions have recognized the dilatory effect time has on our spiritual development. If this is so, how have we become so hypnotized by the effect of time? To answer this question, we need to explore the nature of the body/mind/spirit. When we examine the body in relation to time, we see that it is only capable of experiencing and learning in a linear fashion. The spirit by nature is timeless, but the psyche or mind has the possibility of flowing between both worlds. Due to our physical constitution, it is difficult to remain identified with spirit for a very long time.

To further understand our obsession with temporalities and how they affect our development, we need to review the passage of a human being through time and our attraction to its various elements. Children find it easy to live in the moment because in actuality we are all born in this condition, much like an animal who lives only for the present. As we progress through life's sequence of events, we begin to dwell on the past and ponder about the future. Soon we are caught in the web of time, experiencing guilt complexes about the past, and fear about the future. At other times, we might be caught reminiscing about happy events in the past, or anticipating pleasurable future events. All this ruminating, over the past or the future, leads in only one direction - illusion, and toward the creation of illusory thought crystals. When we are not in the present, we are not in reality. We are not seeing and experiencing life as it really is. As we mature and develop greater conscious awareness, we can then regain our childlike sense of awe in the present moment. Gnostic or "knowing", confidence replaces false hope, and we then move to a higher level of being, no longer in the moment in a naive animal way, but with true knowledge of who we really are. For when we finally mature, hopefully, "selflessness (will have) put a stop to the positive egotism of complacent reminiscence, and the negative egotism of remorse," as Huxley so aptly put it. Thus we will no longer be dwelling in either our positive or negative mental tapes, but living in the eternal moment.

The importance of being conscious in the eternal moment has implications on a universal level as well as on the personal level. Historically, it is clear that political and religious philosophies which are least concerned with events in time, which hold to an eternity - philosophy, are also the most peaceful and non-violent such as Buddhism, Hinduism, and Quakerism in the West. By contrast the Judaic, Christian and

Islamic traditions have all been obsessed with events in time. Whereas eternity philosophies worship God as spirit for its own sake, the time-oriented

philosophies and religions pray to God to help them reach their temporal ends. The focus is on creating an ideal situation or environment off in the distant future, and time-oriented devotees have been willing to kill and maim to get it. In ancient times blood sacrifices provided the needed offering to a God considered to be a destroyer as well as a creator, as the concept of God was then related to the actual creative and destructive patterns in the form of sacrifice to political and religious ideals.

From the above examples, we can see the importance inherent in waking up to the present moment. The global implications are obvious, as well as the personal, for in the end, the only place whence change can occur is in the present moment. The present moment is the only point from which you can act or change anything. All else is an illusion. In this moment lies our power and our possibilities.

> *Whoever builds a house of happiness*
> *for the future*
> *Builds a prison in the present*
>
> *Octavio Paz*

Being in the Moment

Perform this exercise with open or closed eyes. Sit or lie in a relaxed position. Begin by taking nice long slow deep breaths, finally allowing your breath to return to normal. While continuing to follow your breath, observe your mind. Allow all of your thoughts and feelings to flow through unhindered. Refrain from judging. The act of observation may actually cause your mind to "stop", or slow down. When it begins to flow again, notice just how many thoughts are concerned with past or future considerations. Continue to bring yourself back into the present moment.

It is recommended that you perform this exercise almost anywhere and at anytime: while walking, performing simple tasks, in waiting rooms, etc.

Exercise #2:

Creating Cause

List all of the major accomplishments and happenings in your life. Examine them to determine how you were drawn toward them. Did you really "decide" to create those realities? If so, what caused you to make the decisions leading up to these accomplishments? Examine your motivations. Just what is it that drives you to be who your are?

Chapter Ten

Journey into Non-Causal Joy

Until now we have focused on some of the negative aspects of being too overly attached to one's belief systems. We have seen the damage caused by religiously and politically provoked wars, and most of all we have examined how our own attachments to certain judgements, mold and define our very behavior.

On the positive side, relating closely with another person or others will help to make us feel more connected with the planet at large and leave us feeling more fulfilled. If we are too attached to, or identified with our surrounding environment, (friends, career, etc.), it will keep us bound in an illusory state. What is important is that we don't become so identified, that we might feel we cannot live without them. To love someone dearly, yet without attachment, so that they are free to come and go at will and to do whatever they need to fulfill themselves, is the true test of the human being. To love without attachment is a real challenge. To love without taking the other for granted is also a real discipline for most.

If we really want to lead a life with full conscious awareness, and really become one with the present moment, we must leave behind our various attachments and dependencies, and accept full responsibility for our life, with all that that entails. We need to be aware that as we shed these attachments, and hidden subconscious patterns, our suppressed emotions may at last rise to the surface, bringing up pain or fear from long buried memories. Only by facing all of our various aspects will we finally be set free.

In the beginning, when we first come into the world, the creation of an identity is necessary. The mind needs a framework from which to operate, so it creates an identity to give itself a structure. The structures inherent in a certain identity provide us with the opportunity to learn specific lessons, and expeience reality in a certain way relative to our identity. Like an action on stage, we take on a certain role in the theater of life and, through this role, we sample a broad spectrum of experiences, ranging from joy through suffering, loneliness through intimacy, and birth through death. We get to experience all of the ups and downs in this game of life; however, we usually forget that in truth we are really only playing a temporary role. In addition, we often continue to play an old part when we are long overdue to switch roles. For instance, the theater of life may be presenting a comedy, yet we may still be stuck in the role of the tragic hero. At different times in our lives we take on a variety of identities in order to learn lessons corresponding to each unique role, and to discover certain truths.

The flavor of the roles we take on in life are predominantly influenced by our parents. As children, we identify most with our parents; we absorb their identities and take on their behavior patterns, almost as if by osmosis. They point the way for us in life, and are our first real mirrors of experience. Our psyche is very much formed by their example, and it is through them that we learn how to react to the various situations which life brings our way. In effect, they share their knowledge of survival techniques, and teach us the way to get along in the world. For the duration of our childhood we are completely dependent on them; they feed us, house us, and provide us with basic security. As children we never question their actions, because they guarantee our survival.

Children learn by imitation. For better or worse, we continue to imitate our parents behavior patterns long after we have become adults. By adolescence, the learning process is pretty much complete and it is time to start on our own path. If the learning process has been stunted, or if we have been traumatized during any crucial stage of our childhood development, we will tend to carry these stunted aspects into our adult lives. One of the consequences of this is that we tend to look for a partner who is similar to the parent of the opposite sex in order to continue old and familiar behavior patterns. For example, a woman whose mother tended to play the victim role and whose father was a rescuer type, will tend to look for a partner who will also play out the dominant rescuer type. This example illustrates clearly how polarized identities create codependency patterns. We generally tend to seek out relationships with people who play out the shadow aspect of our own active role. Even rebellion against parental authority, which is shown by many adolescents, indicates a clear identification with the parents. Whenever we resist any role, it is a sure sign that we are just as controlled by it, if not more so, than if we identify directly with it and play it out accordingly. In effect, all young people who leave home in a rebellious mood, and play out the opposite of their parents' desires out of spite, have never left the prison of dependency. Blaming parents for their mistakes does not set us free. They themselves were conditioned, and took on the patterns of their parents. They did the best that they could with their level of knowledge. No one, not even our parents, consciously tries to hurt anyone. All suffering and even "evil" seeming behavior is a result of total ignorance and unconsciousness. If people were conscious of the divine law of cause and effect, we would not see so many outward forms of violence in this world.

The age-old unconscious patterns of the past must finally be broken; we must be healed of our past misunderstandings so that we can regain our true center and reclaim our own authority. The key to freedom lies not in blame, but in forgiveness. If we release our past conditioning and let go of our expectations for the future, we can then bring our relationships into the present. This might at first seem risky, as it could bring up surprises we might not feel prepared for, or it could make us feel vulnerable. At the same time, all we could really lose is a fresh new vibrancy and aliveness to being. It is we who must decide to take that risk.

Over the course of a lifetime, it is essential to try on a variety of identities and behaviors without being attached to them, because each one teaches its own lesson. None is really any better than another. Only in this way, with true flexibility, can we discover our limitations and go beyond them. Polarized identities which form the roots of co-dependeny habits, such as victim/rescuer, receiver/giver, strong/weak, ultimately need to be neutralized in order to break through the walls of conditioning. When we focus on and then experience only one side of a polarity, we reduce our infinite potential to the level of a robot who can only play his programmed part. In order to be really free to choose our own roles in life, it is necessary to neutralize not only our attachment to the identity we are actively expressing, but also its polar opposite which is hidden in the shadows of our mind. As we more readily accept all of the various aspects of our being, and integrate them with our experience, the more will we come in contact with the absolute, where duality ceases to exist, and identities fade away.

Any discussion on identities could not be complete without considering one important factor: The self, when it is just one self among otherselves, is a mere limited phenomenon. When we focus on the concept of a self, we are creating further separation of ourselves from the absolute or divine wholeness. Once we identify even with the concept of self, we have then created one more identity and planted further limitation on the path to wholeness. Therefore, ultimately we must even neutralize our concept of Core Self, higher-self, or whatever self we imagine we are striving toward.

Every individual is in every moment in total contact with universal knowledge. It is up to each one of us to strip the veils from blocked consciousness so that we might tune in and reap its abundance. We can not nor should we, wait for others to do it. We only have one chance ever, and that is NOW. When we finally integrate the fact that we are the only true source of our experience, we will also realize that we are also the only ones who can be responsible and committed to really deep change in ourselves.

By expanding our consciousness, we also expand the consciousness of the earth, through the effect of morphic resonance. In other words, as more people concern themselves with the development of consciousness, and take the first bold steps to break the chains that bind us, those that follow will generally have an easier time of it, because the knowledge and experience the path breakers have already gleaned gets passed into the human energy field. Later, others can tap into this living field of knowledge, and speed up their own work on the path to wholeness. Thus it is heartening to know that our own hard efforts will benefit not only ourselves, but many others down the line.

When we neutralize our identities, and behavior and reactive patterns, we effectively dissolve layer upon layer of crystallized thought forms, which may actually be lodged in the cellular structure of the body in the form of melanin protein complex. Both endothermic and exothermic reactions often happen in the body during the dissolving process offering signals which verify the clearing procedure. As this process proceeds, we shed our familiar mental framework, and leave behind the normal signposts of our existence. We move into the vast unknown, which can at first be frightening, but which rewards us finally in our new found freedom. We now surrender to both the negative and positive aspects of life, and enjoy being a fully realized human being. Finally we have thrown away the crutches of our thought forms, and are able to stand on our own two feet. From this moment, we can then direct the game of life.

The more neutral (unconditional) we become, the less we tend to refuse the negative or unpleasant experiences. At a certain point, we begin to accept both the "negative" and "positive" experiences of life as one cyclical flow in the river of life. A non-causal joy then results, as we are no longer attached to having certain types of pleasurable events create our happiness. In addition, so-called "negative" experiences then become a catalyst to the development of a deeper inner power. When we open and surrender to all forms of experience, the universal knowledge then begins to flow unhindered through us. A participant of the Core Empowerment Training described such an experience: "After the first weekend of the training, I started working with one of the exercises I had learned. I began by dissolving some of the thought crystals I had about myself. After completing a few processes, I began to fall asleep, when all of a sudden I noticed a change in my body. I felt all of my bodily tension suddenly disappear. I felt very light, as if I had turned transparent. The most powerful feeling overcame me, as if boundless love and knowledge had permeated every cell of my body. I could feel this energy pulsing through every part of my body. Soon it seemed as if I had become a vibrant gridwork of pulsating light. At the same time, I was very peaceful and felt totally protected in this light. I felt as if there was no more separation between myself and the universe. This sensation may have lasted about ten minutes. Even after the experience, I felt like something was permanently changed on a physical level. I felt a new quality or different sense about my body."

When we release much of the cellular blockage due to thought crystallization, we begin to feel a sense of non-causal joy, which is not nourished by material things or outer stimuli, but by direct experience of the essence of our being.

In this century we have used our minds to discover the secrets of the material universe. Now we can use it to explore the infinite dimensions of our consciousness. The quality of our consciousness determines the quality of our life now and in the future. The way we and the earth will develop, lies partly in our hands. When we bring all our thoughts, motives, feelings, and actions into the light of consciousness, our experiences will change. We can strip away our past conditioning and make a decision to be responsible and accept our freedom. This is our choice. Each of us contributes in every moment to the creation of the universe. To do this in a conscious and responsible way is the challenge of our time.

Let us begin - NOW!

*Don't think! Thinking is the enemy
of creativity. It's self-conscious,
and anything self-conscious is
lousy. You can't try to do things.
You simply must do things.*

Ray Bradbury

Exercise #1:

Examining Co-Dependency

Review your previous relationships with members of the opposite sex. List them on paper. Note any similarities in the relationship between your parents, and the relationship between you and your parent of the opposite sex, or with your current or previous relationships with members of the opposite sex. Notice common patterns in all of these relationships which have been repeated quite often.

Exercise #2:

Mirror Exercise

Find a comfortable sitting position and begin by taking a few deep breaths to relax both your body and mind. During this exercise you should act as a totally passive observer of your environment. Imagine that you are a thoughtless mirror merely reflecting its surroundings. As you sit, allow yourself to observe without reacting, without "doing", without changing anything. Allow yourself to "be" as a mirror - simply a reflection of the objects around you.

The Gratitude Walk

Take a 30 minute meditation walk and say "thank-you" to everything you see, hear, and experience. Greet whatever appears internally or externally, and consciously say Thank You! Develop a feeling of gratitude even for those experiences you tend to judge as uncomfortable or "negative", because every experience is an opportunity for growth and learning.

Glossary

absolute -
refers to the divine aspect of the universal whole, which is free from all qualification or restriction

attachment -
to be bound by personal ties; to be connected to something or someone by one's desire for affection or regard

body electronics -
a system of body work put together by John Ray, utilizing release points, and heightened nutrition, to clear thought crystals

collective unconscious
refers to the unified aspect of the entire human unconscious, which we all tap into

conditioned response -
a set pattern of behavior which has been patterns modified by one stimulus and is generally repeated when exposed to similar stimuli

"conscious"-
when used in quotation marks we are using the word in its usual sense, which refers to our normal mental state when we are awake and moving through the daily patterns of our lives. We are actually going through most of our activities in a very robotic way, pre-programmed by past experience, thus asleep.

conscious -
refers to when we are truly awake and aware in the present moment

conscious mind -
perceives senses such as sound, smell, taste, sight, language, ideas

dis-ease -
an alteration of the living body that impairs its functioning due to it being "ill at ease."

Such a state creates a health challenge for growth and learning.

duality -
the condition of having a twofold aspect or nature

ego -
the main identity we have created of ourself

identity -
to associate oneself as an intrinsic part of something or someone

intellect -
involves our capacity for rationalization and logic; can operate unconsciously or can be used for conscious creation

morphic field -
an ordered region of space which contains a certain resonance of coded knowledge or memory, which resonates to others of a similar nature containing a similar frequency

personality -

is composed of the many I's which make up

each individual's own distinct character

polarity -
the condition of having two poles with opposite vibratory frequencies

polarized identity -
refers to the duel aspect of identity. Humans tend to identify with one side of an opposing identity and remain unconscious of the presence of its polar opposite.

"pushing buttons' -
to create a reaction in another by stimulating one of their vulnerable spots; to challenge someone's Achilles heel.

shadow -
refers to the unconscious opposite of the polarized identity to which we are currently attached

subconscious -
mental activities which exist just below the threshold consciousness

thought crystal -
a judgement or belief which has become crystallized on

both a mental and physical level, which causes us to react to life's circumstances in a predetermined way.

time space continuum -
mental level where all knowledge is accessed

unconscious mind -
takes in all information even while in a coma, or asleep and stores it for life

Introduction to Checklists

The first two checklists are designed to help you take stock of your present life situation. The first checklist was formulated to help point you in the direction of your most predominant patterns so that you may become more aware of them in your everyday life situations. Keeping a journal of your progress each evening is very helpful in bringing these patterns to even greater conscious awareness. The second checklist is intended to help you review your achievements to date, in order to better assess your present quality of life, and to note which areas might need more effort.

The third checklist was created as a guide to help you make decisions and set goals, and formulate steps to reach your goals. Take some time to go through all three checklists. They will help show you more clearly where you presently are in the flow of your life, and help you to set your course for the future.

Personal Growth Checklist

When we observe ourselves honestly, we find that we react to circumstances according to well defined patterns. They may be thought patterns, emotional patterns, behavioral patterns, or combinations of all three. The following checklist will help you notice the recurring patterns in you life, and bring you in touch with areas where growth and awareness are needed.

Find which word most accurately describes the frequency with which you fall into the following patterns. Score yourself according to the
columns provided:

Thought Patterns

Are you ....?

_____ Worrying
_____ Cynical
_____ Pessimistic
_____ Optimistic
_____ Unrealistic (Exaggerating "Good" or "Bad")
_____ Overcritical of Self
_____ Overcritical of Others
_____ Prone to fault finding
_____ Nit-Picking
_____ Indecisive
_____ Needing to control other people
_____ Needing to control situations
_____ Needing to be right
_____ A person who dwells obsessively
_____ on one thought or theme
_____ Unforgiving
_____ A victim of circumstance
_____ Greedy
_____ Loving
_____ Not good enough
_____ Feeling helpless
_____ Doubting

_____ *Fill in any patterns*
_____ *which*
_____ *have been omitted:*

0-Never **1**-Seldom **2**-Occasionally **3**-Frequently **4** -Almost Always

Emotional Patterns

Are you ....?

_____Enthusiastic

_____Lethargic

_____Anxious

_____Irritable

_____Angry

_____Resentful

_____Fearful of others

_____Fearful of authority figures

_____Fearful of close relationships

_____Fearful of being alone

_____Phobic

_____Fearful of dying

_____Filled with grief

_____Dejected

_____Sad

_____Lonely

_____Guilty

_____Without hope

_____Passive

_____Aggressive

_____Emotionally numb

_____ (other)

_____ (other)

_____ (other)

0-Never **1**-Seldom **2**-Occasionally **3**-Frequently **4** -Almost Always

Behavior Patterns

Are you......?

Overly addicted to:

_____ Alcohol
_____ Coffee
_____ Black tea
_____ Cola
_____ Chocolate
_____ Tobacco
_____ Sugar
_____ Street Drugs
_____ Sex

Behavior Patterns

Are you......?

An habitual:

_____pleaser
_____ "motor mouth"
_____over eater
_____exhibitionist
_____flirt
_____macho bully
_____martyr
_____depressive
_____liar
_____loser
_____oversleeper
_____Insomniac
_____"Slob"
_____Compulsively neat and tidy

_____ Do you recognize in yourself any
_____ other habitual or compulsive patterns
_____ such as constantly falling in and out
_____ of love, getting married and divorced,
_____ etc.?

0-Never **1**-Seldom **2**-Occasionally **3**-Frequently **4** -Almost Always

Achievements Checklist

After completing the Personal Growth Checklist, take time to review the areas which need more growth and awareness. The following list will help you review your current and past achievements in the following areas:

1. Spiritual
2. Happiness
3. Family life
4. Other close reationships
5. Education
6. Professional or career
7. Financial
8. Health

After taking time to list your achievements on paper, add any notes or comments which might help you to assess your current position.

Decisions and Goals Checklist

After balancing the information from the Personal Growth Checklist with all of your achievements, you should now turn your attention to the future. In each of the eight areas of achievement, what are your goals? If it takes time to decide, take that time. NOW DECIDE. List your goals. Do not proceed until you have done this!

You now have your goals listed in front of you. Are you TOTALLY WILLING TO COMMIT YOURSELF TO TAKING THE STEPS TO REALIZE YOUR GOALS?

If you are not yet ready to make such a commitment in any area, please STOP. Cross that "Goal" off your list. NOW.

Any "Goal" that is not accompanied by a clear commitment to taking the necessary steps for its achievement, remains nothing but a fantasy, AND THAT FANTASY WILL DRAIN YOUR PSYCHIC AND CREATIVE ENERGY FASTER THAN YOU REALIZE. If this has been an habitual pattern in your life already, you will recognize this truth. Is this true of you? Whether it is or not, is of no consequence at this moment. What does matter is your willingness to make a commitment for change. RIGHT NOW! What you do now affects your whole future.

Take some time to decide now exactly what you want in your life and set your goals accordingly. Once you are clear on your choices in each of the categories, take the time then to plan certain steps which will help you reach these goals.

In some cases you may see clearly the steps which are needed to achieve your goal. If you cannot see all of the steps involved, you can still commence your journey by just listing the first one or two. By committing yourself to your goals and then actually pursuing them physically, you will cause the latter steps to reveal themselves of their own accord and in the proper time. Goethe described the importance of committing oneself to a goal or plan. He made it clear that by making a firm decision, providence itself would then be moved. All sorts of things would occur to help a person which would otherwise not have occurred. Indeed, a whole stream of events would issue from a decision, raising in one's favor all manner of unforeseen incidents and meetings and material assistance which most people could not ever dream

could even happen to them. Thus he stated, "Whatever you can do or dream you can, begin it! Boldness has genius, magic and power in it. Begin it now."

At this point you have your goals, you have your willingness, and you now have your commitment. All that remains before you can set this powerful enterprise in motion is a simple formulation of your first steps toward each of your goals.

How many steps do you need? Just one will suffice, or it may be appropriate to list more than one step for each of your goals. THE IMPORTANT STEP IS THE FIRST STEP. Whether you have steps two, three or four clearly in your mind does not matter here.

Take up your pen and, giving yourself all the time you need, decide on your first steps and list them.

Goals

1. Step 1 _____
   Step 2 _____
   Step 3 _____

2. Step 1 _____
   Step 2 _____
   Step 3 _____

3. Step 1 _____
   Step 2 _____
   Step 3 _____

4. Step 1 _____
   Step 2 _____
   Step 3 _____

5. Step 1 _____
   Step 2 _____
   Step 3 _____

6. Step 1 _____
   Step 2 _____
   Step 3 _____

7. Step 1 _____
   Step 2 _____
   Step 3 _____

8. Step 1 _____
   Step 2 _____
   Step 3 _____

Now review your commitment and take that step.
Bon Voyage

ADDRESSES AND
SOURCES OF SUPPLY
Fragrances, Gemstones, Herbs
Books and Cassettes

WHOLESALE

Contact with your business name,
resale number or practioner license.

LOTUS LIGHT
PO Box 1008 CD
Silver Lake, WI 53170
414/889-8501
Fax 414/889-8591

RETAIL

LOTUS FULFILLMENT SERVICE
33719 116th Street, Box CD
Twin Lakes, WI 53181

I CHING
New Systems, Methods, and Revelations

by Angelika Hoefler

$12.95; 185 pp.; paper; ISBN: 0-941524-37-X

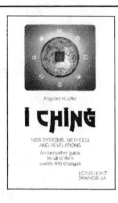

Innovative work on the I Ching, presenting new insights into the use of traditional forecasting tool, making it accessible to the modern reader. Beautifully designed including a meditation drawing for each Hexagram created by the British artist Terry Miller.

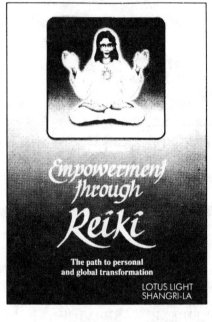

BESTSELLER:

Dr. Paula Horan

Empowerment Through Reiki

The path to personal and global transformation - a handbook

Length: 192 pages
Price: $14.95
Beautifully illustrated
Size: 18cm x 12 cm
ISBN: 0-941524-84-1

ENCHANTING SCENTS

by Monika Junemann

$9.95; 123 pp.; paper; ISBN: 941-524-36-1

The use of essential oils and fragant essences to stimulate, activate and inspire body, mind and spirit.

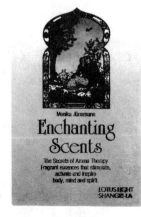

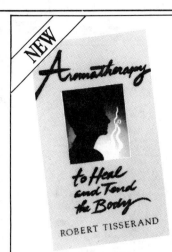

NEW

AROMATHERAPY
To Heal and Tend the Body
by Robert Tisserand   ISBN: 0-941524-42-6
224 pp.; 5½ x 8½; paper; $9.95

The use of aromatic oils to soothe both physical and psychic disorders was recognized in early Egypt and has been rediscovered as a pleasant treatment for a wide range of ailments. The therapeutic properties of the essential oils, together with the relaxation induced by the massage, have been found particularly helpful for stress-related problems. Robert Tisserand's first book, *The Art of Aromatherapy* has become a classic text.

COSMO-BIOLOGICAL BIRTH CONTROL

by Shalila Sharamon & Bodo Baginski
Foreword by Johannes Christ, M.D.

$14.95; 240 pp.; paper; ISBN: 0-941524-82-5

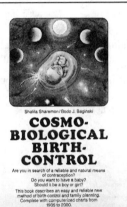

This book describes an easy and reliable new method of birth-control and family planning. Complete with computerized charts from 1935 to 2000.

For the first time, birth-control is evaluated from the interaction of the personal cycle with the cosmic cycles and the book explains why traditional "rhythm method" techniques are insufficient to either avoid or ensure pregnancy.

THE CHAKRA HANDBOOK
By Sharamon & Baginski

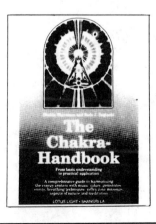

This is the definitive handbook on the Chakras. Their form, color, seed letters sounds etc. and techniques for opening their action.

$14.95; 192 pp; ISBN 0-941524-85-X

CHAKRA ENERGY MASSAGE

By Marianne Uhl

$9.95; 128 pp.; paper; ISBN: 0-941524-83-3

Spiritual evolution into the subconscious through activation of the energy points of the feet.

This book introduces the concept of opening the subtle energy centers of the body through use of foot reflexology.

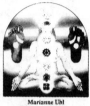

Marianne Uhl

CHAKRA ENERGY MASSAGE

Spiritual evolution·
into the Subconscious
through activation
of the energy points of the feet

LOTUS LIGHT
SHANGRI-LA

SECRETS OF PRECIOUS STONES

by Ursula Klinger Raatz

$9.95; 185 pp.; paper; ISBN: 0-941524-38-8

A guide to the activation of the seven human energy centers using gemstones, crystals and minerals.

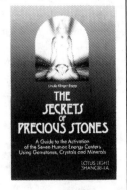

Ursula Klinger Raatz

THE SECRETS OF PRECIOUS STONES

A Guide to the Activation
of the Seven Human Energy Centers
Using Gemstones, Crystals and Minerals

LOTUS LIGHT
SHANGRI-LA